Pycnogenol®
for
Superior Health

Science uncovers the reason why nature's most amazing antioxidant is improving millions of lives

RICHARD A. PASSWATER, Ph.D.

Printed by McCleery and Sons Publishing
3303 Fiechtner Dr SW, Ste 100 • Fargo, ND 58103
800-972-3114 • www.jmcompanies.com

The information contained in this book is based upon the research and personal and professional experiences of the author. They are not intended as a substitute for consulting with your physician or other health care provider. Any attempt to diagnose, prevent and treat an illness should be done under the direction of a health care professional.

The publisher does not advocate the use of any particular health care protocol, but believes the information in this book should be available to the public. The publisher and author are not responsible for any adverse effects or consequences resulting from the use of any of the suggestions, preparations, or procedures discussed in this book. Should the reader have any questions concerning the appropriateness of any procedure or preparation mentioned, the author and the publisher strongly suggest consulting a professional health care advisor.

Pycnogenol® is a registered trademark of Horphag Research, Ltd. Pycnogenol® French maritime pine bark extract is protected by U.S. patent numbers 4,698,360 and 5,720,956.

International Standard Book Number: 0-9712027-3-7

Printed in the USA.

CONTENTS

Introduction

1. An Overview of Pycnogenol® 1
2. The History of Pycnogenol® 13
3. Pycnogenol®:
    The Super antioxidant and More 21
4. Protecting the Heart and Circulation 33
5. Pycnogenol® Against
    Cancer and Other Degenerative Diseases. 49
6. Effects on Aging, Athletic
    Performance, Weight Control
    and Healthy Lifestyle. 59
7. Effects on Varicose Veins Edema,
    "Economy-Class Syndrome," Bruises and
    Venous Health 65
8. Eye Health 71
9. Effects on Sexual Function, Fertility,
    PMS and Menstrual Disorders. 75
10. Effects on Allergies 79
11. Attention Deficit Hyperactivity
    Disorder (ADHD). 81
12. Skincare and Cosmetics 87
13. How to Use Pycnogenol® 93
14. Conclusion 97

    Glossary 99
    References 101
    Suggested Readings 107
    Index 109

INTRODUCTION

If you could take a single natural product to protect and improve your cardiovascular and systemic (entire) circulation system and reduce your risk of heart disease, would you? If you could take a single natural product to reduce inflammation, which aggravates arthritis as well as many other conditions, would you? If you could protect your skin against sun damage including wrinkling and hyper-pigmentation, would you? If you could take a single natural dietary supplement that would reduce your risk of more than 60 diseases and improve your immunity to protect you against germ diseases, allergy and cold symptoms – would you? Of course you would. Any reasonable person would, provided he or she is aware of the strong scientific background of this single natural product.

The one natural product that offers all of these benefits, and more, is an extract from the bark of French Maritime Pine trees. It's called Pycnogenol® (pronounced pick-nah-jeh-nol), and a growing body of scientific research and physicians' experiences shows that it can have a profoundly important effect on health.

Pycnogenol® works for a number of reasons. First, it's a natural complex of several antioxidants—that is, substances that protect your body from free radicals and the ravages of the aging process. Second, it has unique compounds that have specific interactions with several body systems. Third, it contains many of the beneficial compounds found in fruits and vegetables, but it concentrates them so you benefit from higher potencies. Pycnogenol® bears some similarities to the many natural herbal remedies sold, but it has a long track record of exceptional safety.

Pycnogenol® has several key actions when consumed:

* It protects against dangerous molecules known as free radicals,
* which speed up the aging process.
  and set the stage for heart disease, cancer and more than 60 other diseases.
* It strengthens blood vessel walls, protects the linings of blood vessels and reduces edema.
* It improves circulation and helps keep blood cells slippery so that they don't cause the blood clots that result in heart attacks.
* It protects us against stress.
* It boosts immunity.
* It helps relax blood vessels, thereby improving blood circulation and helping to normalize blood pressure.
* It reduces inflammation and helps restore and maintain joint flexibility.
* It eases hay fever and allergies.
* It reduces menstrual disorders.
* It helps keep skin smooth and youthfully flexible.
* It counteracts abnormal pigmentation of the skin.
* It helps protect against the complications of diabetes such as retinopathy.

* It improves learning ability and memory retention.
* It reduces the risk of cataracts.
* It improves healing.
* It can help to overcome attention deficit hyperactive disorder (ADHD, or hyperactivity).

In the first two chapters of *Pycnogenol® for Superior Health*, I describe exactly what Pycnogenol® is, how it is prepared, and a little about its history. I also provide an overview of its health benefits and explain why it does so many good things for health. You'll learn a lot of new, unfamiliar terms, but I will explain exactly what they mean. In subsequent chapters, I delve into the benefits of Pycnogenol® in greater detail and its amazing benefits in circulatory disorders, inflammation, ADHD and other conditions.

Pycnogenol® is a unique supplement. Although many different companies sell Pycnogenol®, it comes from only one source. The makers of some other products may claim similar benefits to Pycnogenol® but, again, there is only one product—patent protected—that comes from French Maritime pine trees, which makes it unique.

Sit back for a few minutes and read how Pycnogenol® can help bring you superior health.

CHAPTER 1

An Overview of Pycnogenol®

A book such as *Pycnogenol® for Superior Health* often begs as many questions as it answers. What exactly is this oddly named supplement? What can it do for your health? How does it work? This chapter answers many of these questions and provides an overview of this remarkable supplement.

Q. What is Pycnogenol® and why is it unique?

A. Pycnogenol® (pronounced pick-nah-jeh-nol) is a dietary supplement-that is, a nutrient or group of nutrients that comes in tablet, capsules or sachets. Pycnogenol® is a complex of several water-soluble, highly bioavailable, antioxidant nutrients extracted from a particular species of Maritime Pine tree (*Pinus maritima* or *Pinus pinaster*, sub-species *atlantica*) found in southwestern France. Many of the nutrients in Pycnogenol® are bioflavonoids, a beneficial group of compounds found in plants. Pycnogenol® contains several classes of bioflavonoids, particularly procyanidins. Some of these bioflavonoids are very simple small molecules. Other bioflavonoids in Pycnogenol® are composed of larger molecules. In addition, there are also several "organic acids," also called fruit acids, found in Pycnogenol®. These are all natural antioxidants.

Q. What does the word "pycnogenol" mean"

A. "Pycnogenol" is a name coined to reflect that many of the nutrient bioflavonoids in Pycnogenol® are made by Nature by joining together smaller bioflavonoids. The larger bioflavonoids are called oligomeric procyanidins which are formed when Nature joins together two or more of the smaller bioflavonoids catechin and/or epicatechin. Chemists call this process "condensation reactions," The word "pycnogenol" was taken from Greek root words that suggest that this blend of bioflavonoids contains large molecules which have been joined together from small molecules."

Q. How was Pycnogenol® discovered?

A. Pycnogenol® is best known today as a complex of powerful antioxidant nutrients. Antioxidants are compounds that protect the body against harmful reactions called free radical reactions. Antioxidants and free radicals are explained later. However, Pycnogenol® is much more than a powerful antioxidant.

The concept involving the earliest use for Pycnogenol® was to help the body function with less vitamin C and prevent scurvy when vitamin C sources were low. Pycnogenol® helps the body recycle used vitamin C back into active vitamin C. Thus, whatever vitamin C is available in the body, it will actively function and longer. The original research was designed to learn how a pine bark decoction prepared by North American Indian medicine men helped vitamin C be more effective. In reading the reports of early European explorers of the North American continent, it was learned that they were saved from the vitamin C deficiency disease called scurvy by a decoction containing a small amount of vitamin C from pine tree needles and pine bark.

Later, researchers learned that this decoction worked because the pine bark was rich in nutrients called bioflavonoids.

Q.   What are bioflavonoids?

A.   Bioflavonoids are nutrients that can replace some of the need for vitamin C in some biochemical reactions and thus, save some vitamin C. Early research by Nobel Laureate Dr. Albert Szent-Gyorgyi suggested that bioflavonoids had additional properties that justified them being classified as vitamins. American scientists have rejected this view, but many European scientists believe that bioflavonoids are at least semi-essential and that the vitamin hypothesis merits further study.

Bioflavonoids, often called flavonoids, are a class of thousands of beneficial compounds found in plants. The structures of these antioxidant compounds enables them to easily donate electrons to other molecules. This ability to donate electrons, a type of subatomic particle, is a characteristic of all antioxidants. There are thousands of bioflavonoids existing in nature. Scientists have identified over 4,000 of them but they are sure that there are several thousand more yet to be identified.

Flavonoids are found in fruits, vegetables, nuts seeds, grains, cacao, and in beverages such as tea and wine. Many flavonoids are pigments that provide several fruits with their blue and purple colors and some of the reds and emerald green.

In addition to their antioxidant properties bioflavonoids have a host of other beneficial effects in the body. Studies have shown that bioflavonoids possess antiviral, anti-inflammatory, antihistamine and even anticarcinogenic properties.

Pycnogenol® contains several classes of bioflavonoids, some are very simple molecules called monomers. Consider a monomer as one bioflavonoid unit. Others compounds in Pycnogenol® contain multiples of these units attached together in a specific way. Compounds consisting of two and three units (monomers) are called dimers and trimers respectively. Still larger compounds are present that consist of four to twelve units. These compounds are called oligomers. In addition, there are organic acids of the family often commonly called fruit acids.

Q. What are procyanidins?

A.   Procyanidins (or proanthocyanidins) are the class of bioflavonoids to which Pycnogenol® belongs. About 250 procyanidins have been identified in nature. They were named so because of the blue hue they give to plants ("cyano-" means dark blue). There was a brief attempt to name these compounds "pycnogenols," which means small molecules joined together to make large molecules, but that usage was promptly discarded, and Pycnogenol® is now used solely as a registered trademark to identify the product that is the complex of bioflavonoids from the bark of the French maritime pine tree.

Q. What are organic acids (fruit acids), and what is their role in Pycnogenol®?

A.   The array of organic acids in Pycnogenol® is often overlooked by researchers who concentrate only on the procyanidins. These natural organic acids are potent antioxidants, but they also reduce the constriction of blood vessels and cramping the uterus, which helps maintain normal circulation and reduces some of the discomfort associated with menstrual periods. They also stimulate the transportation of bile from the liver to the gall bladder which helps promote digestion and the elimination of toxins.

Caffeic acid and ferulic acid, two organic acids found in Pycnogenol®, also help reduce the formation of undesirable nitrosamine compounds which can cause cancer. Additionally, Pycnogenol® and caffeic acid helps protect the liver from some toxic solvents and blocks the formation of undesirable leukotrienes which are mediators of allergic reactions. Ferulic acid has significant anti-inflammatory action and improves capillary permeability. These actions are discussed in more detail later in this book.

The importance of the totality of the unique blend of procyanidins and organic acids has been demonstrated by studies in which Pycnogenol® has been chemically divided into smaller portions. While one fraction shows superiority in one action or another, the benefits of the individual fractions never equals the benefits of the complete blend.

The many diverse nutrients in Pycnogenol® result in synergy unmatched by any other known blend of nutrients. The smaller molecules provide antioxidant activity more quickly and can penetrate into smaller cellular compartments, the larger molecules provide a longer-lasting action as well as more diverse actions. Together, this blend provides actions not demonstrated by any other dietary supplement.

Q.   Are the organic or fruit acids of Pycnogenol® found in foods?

A.   The organic acids found in Pycnogenol® are also

6

found in other foods, including various fruits, vegetables, nuts, seeds, and beans. However, nature does
not combine these various fruit acids in the same plant
in the same combination as in Pycnogenol®, nor in
combination with the same procyanidins.

**Q.   Why is it important that the blend of nutrients
in Pycnogenol® be known and consistent from
batch to batch?**

A.   Scientists stress that it is important for products
used clinically be consistent from batch to batch and
year-to-year. Just think of the medical chaos if peni-
cillin tablets had double the amount one time and half
the amount the next. Or if aspirin varied from batch
to batch.

It is difficult to find natural products that are consistent from crop to crop. Wheat and corn vary in the
nutrient content from season to season and from soil
to soil.   Herbs also vary from source to source.
Pycnogenol® is a natural product that comes from a
single species. The bark of the Maritime Pine grows
over the 25-plus year plus lifetime of the tree and var-
ies little in bioflavonoid content. In Contrast to this,
other natural products such as grapes, that vary, as
wines produced from them also do and from region to
region, from crop to crop. Doctors can't conduct mean-
ingful studies with medicines or nutrients that may
have been from a "vintage year" or not.

Besides being from a single species that grows over
decades in the same region, Pycnogenol® is extracted
by a very controlled process and standardized when
dried to a powder to produce a product that is consistent from batch to batch, year to year.

Q. Since there are more than 40 nutrients in Pycnogenol®, what are its bioflavonoid content specifications?

A. Pycnogenol® contains monomeric units of procyanidins such as catechin and epicatechin and the closely related flavone, taxifolin. It contains at least 60-65% oligomeric procyanidins with chain lengths between 2 and 12 monomeric units. Futhermore, it contains fruit acids such as caffeic acid, ferulic acid, gallic acid, coumaric acid, vanillic acid and others.

Q. Where does Pycnogenol® come from?

A. Pycnogenol® is extracted from the bark of pine tree that grows as a monospecies forest in Southwestern France. This area is free from pesticides and herbicides. The maritime pine from Landes de Gascogne is commonly called the French maritime pine tree. Its formal scientific name is the *Pinus pinaster*, subspecies *atlantica*. However, it is also referred to in the scientific literature as Atlantic pine, *Pinus maritima,* Pin des Landes, *Pinus pinaster* Sol., and *Pinus pinaster* Aiton. Regardless of the different names, it is the only species that grows in the 4,000.square-miles (one million hectares) as a forest along the Bay of Biscay (Atlantic Ocean), situated between the vineyards of Bordeaux to the north and the Pyrenees Mountains to the south.

No trees are cut down only for the purpose to produce Pycnogenol®. The bark is a by-product of the lumber and resin industries, but it is of special importance and receives special handling. The bark of the Maritime Pine is thick, dark reddish-brown, and deeply fissured. Its thickness protects the bioflavonoids before the nutrients are extracted. However, it is still important to extract bioflavonoids from the bark within forty-eight hours of cutting down the trees for lumber. It takes about 1000 kilograms of flavonoid-rich Maritime Pine bark to produce one kilogram of Pycnogenol®.

Q.   Whoever heard of nutrients from tree bark? We don't eat tree bark do we?

A.   Well, yes we do eat tree bark when it is necessary, and we also benefit from medicines extracted from tree bark. Many people living in the far north consider pine bark to be the banana of the north because of its non-toxic, moderate nutrient content. The bark is dried and made into a flour to make bark bread. Normally bark is used as an extender for normal bread grains, but bark bread itself is occasionally used to supplement normal diets in northern climates. During times of famine, bark bread becomes a staple. In Finland, during the famines of 1601-1602, 1695-1697, 1867-1868 and 1918, bark bread was often the only available source of food.

As mentioned, bark has been used as herbal medicines. Most people are familiar with the fact that aspirin was first derived from willow bark more than one hundred years ago. The salicylic acid from willow bark was effective against pain, but the derivative, acetylsalicylic acid is more effective. In the early days in the U. S., powdered bark was used on wounds to promote healing and was a basis for cough syrups. In Asia, tree bark extracts were used to treat cardiac arrhythmias (irregular heart beats). In Europe tree bark extracts have been used to treat liver, kidney and skin disorders.

The use of greatest historical interest to the Pycnogenol® story is that of the North American Indians in curing scurvy but that's another story for chapter two.

Q. If the active compounds come from trees, are they not more like herbs than nutrients? What foods contain the active components of Pycnogenol®?

A.   The procyanidins of Pycnogenol® are specific because they come from a unique plant – the French maritime pine — other procyanidins, and the identical monomers and organic acids are found in a broad range of fruits and vegetables. Some are also found in some herbs. Various procyanidins are found in sorghum, avocado, strawberries, bananas, grapes and others. However, nowhere else in nature are the specific procyanidins and the unique blend of bioflavonoid nutrients found. As examples, procyanidins are found in grapes, and caffeic acid and ferulic acid are found in parsley and spinach. Caffeic acid is also found in onions, and ferulic acid is also found in rhubarb and grapes. Gallic acid is found in eggplant and radish.

The purpose of supplementing with Pycnogenol® is not only to upgrade a poor diet, it is to boost your antioxidant defenses and achieve many health benefits not achievable by diet alone. Pycnogenol® can partly compensate for the bioflavonoids and other antioxidants missing in diets low in fruits and vegetables. Few Americans eat the recommended five full servings of fruits and vegetables.

Q. How does Pycnogenol® work?

A.   After seeing the long list of health benefits, you might wonder how could one supplement possibly do so much? Part of the answer is that Pycnogenol® is not just one nutrient. Since it contains so many nutrients, it has several diverse actions. Most of the compounds act chiefly as antioxidants, while others block the actions of undesirable compounds in the body.

Another part of the explanation is that some of the nutrients such as the antioxidants, affect many body systems and thus are factors in preventing many diseases. Antioxidants are involved in reducing the risk of more than sixty diseases. The action of Pycnogenol® in boosting the immune system explains how it increases protection against many infections.

A brief summary of Pycnogenol's® biochemical actions are 1) It terminates free radicals thus protecting cells, 2) It enhances immune function, 3) It binds to the skin proteins collagen and elastin to protect tissue and to seal leaky capillaries, 4) It improves the functioning of blood vessels, large and small, from arteries to the microcirculation of capillaries, and 5) It inhibits tiny blood cells from sticking together to cause circulation problems from heart attacks to strokes to deep vein thrombosis.

Q.   What are the health benefits of Pycnogenol®?

A.   Pycnogenol® helps protect against diseases associated with aging. Many of the health benefits of Pycnogenol® were briefly mentioned in the introduction and will be discussed later in their appropriate chapters. However, the main health benefits are outstanding antioxidant protection against more than 60 diseases including heart disease and stroke, improved circulation as a result of improving both the blood vessels and the blood cells, help in combating the effects of stress and help in maintaining healthy young-performing skin.

In addition, Pycnogenol® even offers some help against the diseases caused by germs as it helps maintain a healthy immune system.

Q. How were so many other health benefits of Pycnogenol® discovered?

A. Pycnogenol® is now known for its strong anti-oxidant effects, but its earlier uses were for other health benefits. Scientists and physicians continually learn of additional health benefits as more and more people use it.

After Pycnogenol® was introduced in Europe as a product to help nourish capillaries (small blood vessels) and skin as suggested by the research on bioflavonoids by Dr. Szent-Gyorgyi, European physicians discovered that Pycnogenol® did much more. With use, it was discovered that Pycnogenol® also was a natural cure for hay fever.

Through the years, research has shown that Pycnogenol® increases capillary resistance by protecting collagen, a ground substance between the cells. This was part of the explanation as to why a pine bark decoction used by the North American Indians cured scurvy. In scurvy, blood leaks out of the capillaries to virtually drown the victims in their own blood. Further research with Pycnogenol® and capillaries confirmed that it improves microcirculation by both improving capillary strength and improving blood cell flexibility. Soon it was also learned that Pycnogenol® improves skin by reducing the degradation of the skin proteins, collagen and elastin.

It was not until 1987 that a patent was issued for Pycnogenol's® strong antioxidant effect that protects so well against harmful free radicals. Since that time researchers in the U. S. became very interested in Pycnogenol®. Beginning in 1995, research reports started appearing by scientists showing that Pycnogenol® regenerates vitamin C, and protects against stress and smoking risk factors involved in heart disease and stroke, reduces stress-induced increases in blood pressure, and improves the immune system.

Q. Is there research to prove Pycnogenol's® health benefits?

A. Definitely. Several animal studies have been carried out, followed by clinical studies conducted by the company that developed the product. There are also several anecdotal reports stemming from thirty years of use in Europe and more than fourteen years (at this writing) of use in the United States. While these are important, what we will be concerned with in this book are the modern studies that have been done with Pycnogenol® and published in the open scientific and medical literatures by scientists throughout the world. I'll describe many of these studies throughout this book.

CHAPTER 2

The History of Pycnogenol®

Researchers now believe that they have traced the origin of Pycnogenol® back to the fourteenth century. Much of the modern research on this antioxidant complex was sparked by accounts of how North American Indians used a pine bark decoction to cure many of Jacques Cartier's explorers of deadly scurvy. In this section, we will recount the historical background and follow that lead to the forefront of modern science. Not only does Pycnogenol® have a long and colorful history, it has proven its value over decades of commercial use with millions of consumers around the world. It has made a significant difference in the health of these people.

Q. How was Pycnogenol® discovered by the western world?

A. Before Pycnogenol® was developed as a dietary supplement, there were reports throughout history of decoctions made from pine bark that healed various ailments. The earliest such reports have been traced back to about 1300. The report that sparked modern research was from Jacques Cartier's French expedition in 1535 to find a northwest passage to China. During the winter, the expedition became prisoners of the frozen Hudson Bay and had to stop at the North American Indian villages of Stadacona and Hochelaga.

Because they had to spend the entire winter there, they exhausted their supply of fresh foods. The explorers soon developed scurvy, a severe deficiency of vitamin C.

Scurvy had already killed twenty-five members of the expedition, and fifty more were seriously ill by the time Cartier befriended a local Native American, Chief Domagaia. The chief prepared a decoction from what was described as a conifer believed to have been pine, but could have been a tree commonly called Anneda or arbor vitae. The bark and needles were boiled to make a tea that was drunk several times a day. The men recovered within a week or two after beginning the treatment. The tea worked because the needles contained traces of vitamin C and the bark provided large quantities of bioflavonoids, stop the bleeding of the gum and strengthens the tissue and the blood vessels, and increase the bio-availability of vitamin C.

Cartier wrote about all this in his Voyages au Canada, published in 1545. An extensive review of the use of pine bark has been written by Dr. G. Drehsen. (Drehsen 1999).

Q. What is scurvy?

A. Scurvy is a disorder that results from a deficiency of vitamin C. It was common to early sailors who explored far from their home ports and, as a consequence, lacked diets rich in vitamin C.

Scurvy develops when there is not enough vitamin C to produce adequate collagen-the protein essential for capillary and skin health. Without enough collagen to form the ground substance that fills the space between cells in the capillary walls, the capillaries leak so badly that they bleed. The symptoms of scurvy begin with muscle pains and weakness leading to total exhaustion with very little effort expended. The joints ache and even minor movement causes breathlessness. The skin becomes sallow and dusky. Deep depression soon sets in. The gums bleed profusely and the teeth fall out. In a matter of a few weeks after the first signs are apparent, the internal bleeding is so severe that it leads to lung and kidney failure and then death.

Q.   Who figured out what Pycnogenol® contains?

A.   Scientists aware of the historical accounts of Cartier's explorers being cured of scurvy became intrigued and wanted to find out why a tree bark extract cured the explorers.

Early research indicated that the vitamin C-like action of pine bark extracts was due to substances in the bark called bioflavonoids. Later, in 1970, with the advent of better analytical instruments and funding from Horphag Research Ltd., using an extract from the bark of the Maritime Pine tree that grows in the Landes de Gascogne in the southwest of France, it was determined that these substances were a defined mixture of organic acids and procyanidins. In 1984, G. Pirasteh, Ph.D., and Peter Rohdewald, Ph.D., identified and quantified most of the ingredients.

Q.   How long has Pycnogenol® been available as a dietary supplement?

A.   Pycnogenol® was introduced as a dietary supplement in the United States in 1987. Since the research supporting the supplement was unknown in the United States, and there are strict regulations against making drug-like claims for dietary supplements, few knew about the health benefits of Pycnogenol®.

Also in 1987, Pycnogenol® was granted a patent in the United States as a novel and powerful antioxidant and free-radical scavenger. At the beginning of the 1990s, the general population was beginning to learn of the health benefits of antioxidants. As more people learned of the antioxidant power of Pycnogenol®, they also learned of its other health benefits.

Pycnogenol® was formally approved as a Food Supplement in the United Kingdom by the Ministry of Agriculture, Fishery and Foods (MAFF) in 1999.

Slowly but surely, Pycnogenol's® benefits became known as one helped person told another, and today it is one of the most popular dietary supplements sold in health foods and drug stores, as well as other channels including the internet.

Q. Do doctors know about the many health benefits of Pycnogenol®?

A. Today, many do. In the 1990s, it was widely recommended by holistic physicians (also referred to as integrative, complementary, orthomolecular or alternative medicine physicians), but was not well known by most of the orthodoxy. Holistic physicians prefer to use safe, natural nutrients when possible because of the additional health benefits and lack of side effects. These physicians attend many nutritional seminars and study nutritional science publications and journals. A large percentage, if not most, of the holistic physicians recommend or prescribe Pycnogenol® because of its proven benefits and their experience in their own practice.

Doctors normally learn of the benefits of drugs from pharmaceutical representatives called "detail" men or women. Although there are no "detail " sales persons to educate the conventional doctors about nutrients as there are for drugs, many conventional doctors have learned about the benefits of Pycnogenol® from the success stories of their patients. Today, many doctors have been introduced to Pycnogenol® by their peers and their patients.

Q. What research has been conducted on Pycnogenol®?

A. Research has been carried out on Pycnogenol® since 1965. However, these data have been retained as unpublished internal research reports of the company who developed the product. Extensive safety studies have been carried out under the direction of Dr. Peter Rohdewald of the University of Muenster in Germany. Past research on capillary health has been conducted by Dr. Miklos Gabor (Gabor *et al.,* 1993) of the Szent -Gyorgyi Medical University in Hungary. Studies on Pycnogenol® protection of skin have been carried out by Dr. Antti Arstila of the University of Jyvaeskylae in Finland (Guochang, 1993)

More recent research has centered on Pycnogenol's® effects on heart disease, the immune system, attention deficit disorder, and Alzheimer's disease. Ronald Watson, Ph.D., of the University of Arizona, Tucson, has been researching Pycnogenol's® action in boosting the immune system, (Cheshier *et al.,* 1996) protection against sunburn (Saliou et al., 2001), improvement of hypertension (personal communication) and protecting against heart disease. (Watson, 1999) Dr. Lester Packer of the University of California, Berkeley, is studying how Pycnogenol® works as an antioxidant, how it protects nerve cells, and how it acts as an anti-inflammatory agent. (see review by Packer *et al.,* 1999)

Dr. Schubert of the Salk Institute has studied how Pycnogenol® helps protect against Alzheimer's disease. Dr. Lau of Loma Linda University has discovered that Pycnogenol® enhances antioxidant defenses of body cells, (Rong *et al.,* 1995) and improves learning ability and memory retention. (Liu *et al.,* 1999)

Dr. Lau and his colleagues have also found that Pycnogenol® compensates for the age-related decline of the immune system. (Liu *et al.,* 1998). They have further shown that Pycnogenol® inhibits generation of inflammatory mediators in the inflammatory cells. (Bayeta and Lau, 2001).

Dr. T. Kohama, a Japanese gynecologist, showed Pycnogenol's® benefits for menstrual disorders. (Kohama and Suzuki, 1999) Dr I. (Ken) Jialal and his colleagues at the University of Texas at Dallas, demonstrated that the blood of volunteers who took Pycnogenol® had a significantly increased antioxidant capacity. (Yang *et al.,* 2001)

Professors Arcangeli and Spartera of the University of Aquila, Italy in independent clinical studies have shown beneficial effects of Pycnogenol® in chronic venous insufficiency. (Arcangeli, 2000; Petrassi *et al.,* 2000) Professor Baleṣtrazzi from the same University showed Pycnogenol's® benefits in diabetic retinopathy. (Spadea and Balestrazzi, 2001)

As the number of scientific publications increase, there will be additional scientists eager to research the health benefits of Pycnogenol®.

Q. Is Pycnogenol® patented?

A. Yes, It Is. Pycnogenol® is patented in the United States, Europe, China and Japan, with several additional patent applications pending in the United States, Japan and China. US patent number 4,696,360 was granted in 1987 for Pycnogenol's® use as a powerful antioxidant and free-radical scavenger. It was issued on October 6, 1987.

Another US patent (5,720,956) was issued on February 24, 1998. It is titled "Method of controlling the reactivity of human blood platelets by oral administration of the extract of the maritime pine (Pycnogenol®) and lists Peter Rohdewald as the inventor and is assigned to Horphag Research. In fact, these patent numbers and/or the name "Horphag" or the logo of the pine tree are cited on the label of the package to assure authenticity of the product.

Q. Is Pycnogenol® trademarked?

A. Yes. The U.S. Patent and Trademark Office issued a trademark to Horphag Research for the name "Pycnogenol®" for dietary and nutritional supplements on May 11, 1993. An official logo depicting a pine tree encircled with the words "Pycnogenol® French Maritime Pine Bark Extract" is often used on products and advertisements.

In addition to the United States, Pycnogenol® is a registered trade name in more than 90 countries of the world including, as examples, Brazil, India, Italy, Singapore, Spain, and UK.

CHAPTER 3

Pycnogenol®:
The Superantioxidant and More!

Free radicals are harmful molecules that damage the body and can lead to more than sixty diseases. As will be explained in later chapters, free radicals are involved in cardiovascular diseases and other chronic degenerative diseases. Free radicals also accelerate the aging process, and as a result are involved in decreasing our defenses against germs. Arthritis, Alzheimer's disease, and Parkinson's disease are also linked to free radicals, and studies indicate that antioxidants likely reduce the risk of these diseases.

As a powerful antioxidant that also helps recharge other antioxidants, Pycnogenol® helps protect us against the damage of free radicals very effectively and thus helps protect us from the more than sixty diseases associated with free radicals.

Q. What is an antioxidant?

A. Oxygen is a very reactive element, which is why it rusts iron, promotes combustion, and supports the life process. Iron and iron-containing objects that are left out in air (which contains oxygen) rust, or as chemists say, "oxidize." The process by which things react with oxygen is called oxidation. A substance that prevents or slows the oxidation process is called an antioxidant. Antioxidants also protect other substances, such as living tissue, against damage caused by oxygen.

In the body, it's important for oxygen to be channeled into the right places and kept away from other places. We don't want oxygen to react with vital cell components. This would damage them much like rust damages iron. In the body, unwanted oxidation of cell components can set the stage for aging, heart disease, cancer and many other chronic degenerative diseases. Antioxidants sacrifice themselves to protect vital components.

Q. What qualifies a nutrient to be called an antioxidant?

A.   To qualify to be called an antioxidant, a few good molecules must protect many, many other molecules by neutralizing bad molecules or fragments of molecules. Our bodies make some antioxidants. However, we are dependent on the diet to supply many antioxidants. Important antioxidant nutrients include vitamins, minerals, amino acids, and coenzymes.

Minerals are not direct antioxidants, but several minerals can become vital components of antioxidant enzymes made by the body. Such minerals include selenium, which is needed to make the antioxidant enzyme glutathione peroxidase; iron, which is needed for catalase; and manganese, copper, and zinc, which are-needed to make superoxide dismutase. (Incidentally, Pycnogenol® contains these minerals).

Sulfur compounds, such as the sulfur-containing amino acids cysteine and methionine, help the body produce the most common antioxidant within cells, glutathione.

Antioxidant coenzymes, such as nicotinamide adenine dinucleotide (NADH), coenzyme Q10 and alpha-lipoic acid, can be made in the body as well as obtained in the diet.

Q: Why does Pycnogenol® qualify to be called a unique antioxidant?

A. Pycnogenol® contains very powerful organic antioxidants such as the relatively large molecules of the procyanidins and the relatively small molecules such as catechin, epicatechin and organic acids. The large array of molecular size in the numerous antioxidants allow antioxidants to reach cell interiors as well as circulate in the blood stream to protect the cell exteriors.

In addition to its antioxidant compounds that have a direct protective factor, Pycnogenol® has an indirect protective effect by improving other antioxidants in the cells.

Not only does Pycnogenol® contain potent organic antioxidants and measurable levels of the inorganic minerals the body needs to build antioxidant enzymes, it is important to note that Pycnogenol® increases the levels of these antioxidant enzymes and related antioxidants inside the cells. Dr. Wei and colleagues have shown that Pycnogenol® can double the concentration of superoxide dismutase, catalase and glutathione. (Wei *et al.*, 1997)

Q. How does Pycnogenol® regenerate, or recycle, other antioxidants?

A. One of the reasons that antioxidants work together synergistically is that some antioxidants can regenerate

24

other antioxidants. As an example, Pycnogenol® can regenerate "used" or "spent" vitamin C, which in turn, can regenerate used vitamin E. (Cossins *et al.,* 1998) This means that Pycnogenol® enables the sparse amounts of vitamin C and vitamin E found in most diets function as if there were higher levels in diet. This is a result of recharging the spent vitamins to work again instead of being removed from the body.

When vitamin E or vitamin C molecules come into contact with free radicals, they donate an electron to the free radical and make it a normal nonreactive molecule. This causes the vitamin E or vitamin C molecule to become a weak free radical. This weak free radical does no harm to the body, but since it has given up an electron itself, it can no longer stop free radical reactions by donating an electron. Thus, the vitamin E radicals or vitamin C radicals are useless and usually the body simply destroys them by breaking them apart into smaller compounds to permit their removal from the body via the kidneys.

On the other hand, if the inactive vitamin C radical comes into contact with one of the bioflavonoids in Pycnogenol®, it can be regenerated back into active vitamin C. Active vitamin C can also regenerate an inactive vitamin E radical back into active vitamin E. This effect of Pycnogenol® is possible because the larger procyanidin molecules in Pycnogenol® stabilize the lifetime of the inactive vitamin C radical so that it doesn't decompose and leave the body, but can last long enough to capture its missing electron from one of the many molecules of the procyanidins.

Q. What is a free radical?

A. You can think of free radicals as biological terrorists. Quite simply, they can be bad for your health.

In chemistry, atoms that often are found grouped together can be called a "radical." This group or radical generally stays together during a chemical reaction and can be transferred from molecule to molecule.

Sometimes during very high energy chemical reactions, radicals can have an electron pulled away, causing the group to temporarily break free from the molecule. When this happens, it is called a "free radical." While this unstable, high-energy fragment is free, its energy forces attract an electron from other molecules. A free radical can pull an electron from most biological compounds, thus restoring its original electron content, but causing the other compound that has lost an electron to itself become a free radical.

This free radical reaction can perpetuate until a key biological molecule becomes permanently damaged. Scientists have estimated that each cell in your body (and you have billions of cells) suffers 10,000 free radical "hits" each day. The amount of damage depends on how well the cell is protected by antioxidants. The higher your levels of antioxidants, the greater the amount of protection.

Q. What are some of the "free-radical" diseases?

A. Free radicals damage cell membranes, cellular proteins, DNA, RNA and other essential body components disrupting normal biochemistry and leading to many diseases. Free radicals can be the sole cause of a few diseases, but more often are involved in the disease process by predisposing the human body to diseases directly caused by other factors. Free radicals also may worsen the conditions and be antagonistic to the healing process.

First, let's look at the health condition or diseases

involving more than one organ. These include aging, including disorders of "premature aging" and immune deficiency of aging; cancer; Inflammatory-immune injury, including nutritional deficiencies, alcohol damage and radiation injury, reproductive disorders, and abnormal sperm morphology.

Then there are the diseases that involve a primary single organ. These include blood cell disorders, including systemic lupus erythematosus and sickle-cell anemia; lung disorders, including asthma, cigarette smoke-induced effects, emphysema, hyperoxia, bronchopulmonary dysplasia, cystic fibrosis, oxidant pollutants, acute respiratory distress syndrome (ARDS); heart and cardiovascular system, including atherosclerosis (via oxidation of LDL), heart attack (acute myocardial infarction via coronary thrombosis via platelet aggregation), endothelial injury, vasospasms, and kidney disorders; —gastrointestinal tract and liver disorders, including hepatitis, Endotoxin liver injury, joint abnormalities including rheumatoid arthritis; brain disorders, including neurotoxins, senile dementia, Parkinson's disease, Alzheimer's disease, stroke (thrombosis in cerebral vessels), cerebral trauma from stroke (hypertensive cerebrovascular injury); eye disorders, including cataract, macular degeneration, ocular hemorrhage, degenerative retinal damage, diabetic retinopathy and photic retinopathy; skin disorders, including melasma (chloasma), sunburn (solar radiation), burn (thermal injury), psoriasis and dental diseases including periodontitis.

There are more, but I think you get the idea.

Q. What makes Pycnogenol® different from other antioxidants?

A. Pycnogenol® is much more than a powerful,

multipurpose antioxidant. It also has strong anti-inflammatory, immune boosting, spasmolytic (anti-spasmodic), and anticoagulant (anti-blood clotting) actions. All of these actions combine to give Pycnogenol® a unique position with significant health benefits not known to be produced by any other antioxidant nutrient.

As far as its antioxidant capabilities go, Pycnogenol® is a very powerful antioxidant that is effective against many types of harmful free radicals. While some antioxidants such as vitamin C or vitamin E destroy several types of free radicals and other reactive oxygen species, Pycnogenol®, with its blend of many different antioxidants, destroys more types of free radicals and reaches more compartments of the body than any other antioxidant nutrient.

In addition, Pycnogenol® helps balance and control the production of nitric oxide, which is a good compound in the artery linings and certain other areas, but can be a very harmful compound otherwise. We will discuss nitric oxide later in the chapter on heart disease.

Q. Is Pycnogenol® the most powerful antioxidant nutrient?

A. It may be, according to the studies by Lester Packer, Ph.D., and his colleagues at the University of California, Berkeley in 1997. (Noda *et al.*, 1997) At least it's the most powerful antioxidant complex that has been widely studied under identical laboratory conditions and reported in the scientific literature.

When the several studies of Pycnogenol's® antioxidant capabilities are considered together, they indicate that Pycnogenol® may be the most powerful scavenger of oxygen free-radicals and nitrogen free radicals, as well as other reactive oxygen species (ROS) and reactive nitrogen species (RNS). (Virgili *et al.,* 1998) Pycnogenol® has been shown to be the strongest hydroxyl free radical and superoxide anion radical scavenger among compounds and extracts tested. (Noda *et al*, 1997)

When Pycnogenol® was patented for its free-radical scavenging effect in 1987, it was described as being many times more powerful than vitamin E and vitamin C. This is certainly true under certain conditions. The specific laboratory test used to make the comparison (called the nitrobluetetrazolium, or NBT, test), however, is only one measure of a compound's antioxidant and free-radical scavenging capabilities. However, this test, which is done in a water-based system, would certainly not be a fair one to use to compare Pycnogenol's® antioxidant properties with vitamin E's, as vitamin E is not soluble in water. Conversely, it would not be fair to test Pycnogenol® directly in a lipid (fatty) system.

When comparing antioxidants, several factors must be looked at. One antioxidant may be better retained in one body organ or system or another. An antioxidant may be more efficient against one type of free radical or another. The only fair way to compare antioxidants is to compare their profiles of actions against various free radicals.

Pycnogenol® has been rated the best of the many antioxidants that Dr. Packer compared for their effectiveness against several free radicals that are present in the body. In those systems in which Pycnogenol® has an effect—which includes many systems important to health—he has found Pycnogenol® to be the most effective of all nutrients he tested.

In a more biologically relevant setting, Dr. M. Chida and his colleagues carried out a study to compare the ability of different antioxidants to protect retinal lipids (fats) from damage by free radicals. He found that Pycnogenol® was far more potent that vitamins C and E, lipoic acid, Coenzyme Q10 and grape seed extract. (Chida *et al.*, 1999)

The point is that there may not be just one antioxidant nutrient that is the best in all possible systems—but Pycnogenol® appears to be the most powerful in the most systems, especially of the systems of major importance, and it definitely should be in everyone's defense against free radicals.

Q. Why is Pycnogenol® such a powerful antioxidant?

A. An important reason why Pycnogenol® is such a potent antioxidant is that it is a natural mixture of several types of antioxidants, so it distributes antioxidant nutrients widely throughout the body.

The Pycnogenol® complex of antioxidants provides compounds of varying sizes that can function effectively in different regions of the body over varying periods of time. The larger procyanidins are very effective in the bloodstream, whereas the smaller flavonoid molecules and organic acids can readily enter cell interiors. The large oligomeric procyanidins have several points in their molecules that can annihilate free radicals. Vitamin E in contrast has only one such point. The free-radical annihilating points are called phenolic groups, and vitamin E is a monophenol whereas Pycnogenol® is a polyphenol.

In addition, the several types of antioxidant compounds in Pycnogenol® make it a multipurpose intracellular and extracellular antioxidant. It protects the cell interiors as well as exteriors and circulates in the bloodstream to destroy free radicals there before they can do damage to body components.

The various nutrients in Pycnogenol® have chemical structures that protect against different types of free radicals. Whereas a single antioxidant compound, such as vitamin E or vitamin C, is protective against a number of free radicals, a mixture of many different types of antioxidants protects against a greater number of types of free radicals. Its unique position is caused by its ability to double the content of antioxidative enzymes inside the cell, in addition to directly neutralise free radicals.

Q. So, if Pycnogenol® is so powerful, do we need other antioxidants?

A. The fact that Pycnogenol® is a powerful and versatile antioxidant does not mean that it is the only antioxidant that you should take as a supplement. Many antioxidant nutrients work together as a team. Some simple antioxidants, such as vitamin C and vitamin E, are essential to life and must be part of the diet to maintain life.

Others, such as coenzyme Q10, alpha-lipoic acid, and NADH, can be made in the body and are not dietary essential even though they are also involved in metabolism. These antioxidant nutrients have specific roles that are not replaced by other antioxidants. However, they can be readily consumed by free-radical reactions, and they are not abundant in the diet.

Pycnogenol® has sparing action on vitamin C and can

regenerate used vitamin C into active vitamin C. (Cossins *et al.,* 1998) Vitamin C can, in turn, recycle used vitamin E into active vitamin E, Vitamin E is fat-soluble and dwells in the body in fat-friendly areas, such as cell membranes and lipoproteins. Vitamin C and the bioflavonoids of Pycnogenol® are water-soluble and dwell in the water-compatible areas such as the bloodstream and cell interiors.

Although Pycnogenol® is not considered to be a dietary essential nutrient, Pycnogenol® should be included in the daily diet because it is a powerful antioxidant that has many additional health benefits.

CHAPTER 4

Protecting the
Heart and Circulation

There are several forms of heart disease, thus there are several causes. Most people think of a heart attack as the end result of heart disease, and most people associate cholesterol with heart disease. In this chapter, we explore the causes of heart disease and other circulatory disorders and discuss the cardiovascular benefits of Pycnogenol®.

Q. What exactly is a heart attack, and what causes it?

A. Atherosclerosis, the medical term for narrowed arteries, does not by itself cause heart attacks. Thrombosis (blood clot) and vasoconstriction (constriction and/or spasm of an artery) are the events that usually precipitate a heart attack.

Narrowed arteries (blood vessels that carry blood from the heart) put the squeeze on blood platelet cells and damage them. Platelet cells are the cells that clump and clot in the blood. If you have a cut, they clot and keep you from bleeding to death. But in blood vessels, platelet aggregation leads to clots that interrupt the flow of blood. Clots can lodge in the narrowed arteries of the heart (coronary arteries) completely shutting off the flow of blood through that artery. When this happens, doctors call it a coronary thrombosis—a blood clot in a coronary artery. Hence, the expression that someone is having a "coronary."

When a blood clot shuts off the flow of blood in a coronary artery, the region of the heart fed by the artery is starved of oxygen and nutrients. The result is the death of these cells, which is called an infarct. This is the classic heart attack, called an acute myocardial (heart) infarction, called AMI for short

Vasoconstriction causes reduced blood flow to the heart by constricting the diameter of the artery. It can even completely shut off an artery and stoop all blood flow.

Q. What are some other common heart diseases?

A. Another common form of heart disease is heart failure, in which the heart is too weak to efficiently pump blood. Usually, the heart enlarges as it tries to compensate for the reduced output. Angina is the pain experienced in the heart when there is not enough blood reaching all parts of the heart during activity. High blood pressure (hypertension) affects arteries and is a risk factor in various forms of heart disease.

Q. How do cholesterol deposits form?

A. The process is very complicated, but it's important to remember that free radicals are involved and that Pycnogenol®, as an antioxidant, is protective. Cholesterol is not soluble in blood, so it is carried in particles called lipoproteins. Two important lipoproteins are low-density lipoproteins (LDL) and high-density lipoproteins (HDL). The cholesterol carried by LDL, often called the "bad cholesterol," is carried to the cells from the liver. The cholesterol carried by HDL is often called the "good cholesterol" as it is being carried away from cells and back to the liver.

Cholesterol deposits form only when LDL becomes damaged by oxidation—that is, by free radicals. It's then called "oxidized LDL." Oxidized LDL can infiltrate the artery wall and initiate a series of events that traps the cholesterol-containing oxidized LDL inside the blood vessel wall. White blood cells, sensing that something is wrong, are attracted to the site and swell, forming what are called "foam cells" which then turn into the lesions commonly called "cholesterol deposits."

Q. How does Pycnogenol® protect against cholesterol deposits?

A. LDL is oxidized only when the amount of antioxidants is insufficient to protect the LDL against oxidation. Studies by Dr. A. Nelson and colleagues in 1998 showed that Pycnogenol® directly protects LDL. (Nelson *et al.,* 1998) However, Pycnogenol® can also indirectly protect LDL. The prime antioxidant that protects LDL is vitamin E. Pycnogenol® can recycle vitamin C, which, in turn, can recycle vitamin E.

Pycnogenol® can also destroy the free radicals before they reach LDL to cause damage. The tendency to form oxidized LDL, and hence the cholesterol deposits (atherosclerosis), is dependent on two factors: the amount of LDL and the balance between antioxidants and free radicals. Both are important but the antioxidant/free radical balance is the more important of the two.

It's also important to recognize that the so-called bad cholesterol, the LDL, is not bad unless it is deprived of antioxidants. LDL is needed to transport fat—soluble antioxidants (such as vitamin E) through the bloodstream, which means it's essential for health. But like the rest of the body, LDL cholesterol also needs antioxidants to stay healthy.

Q. How does Pycnogenol® protect against other causes of heart disease?

A. Cholesterol deposits by themselves don't cause a heart attack. They are a major contributing factor to forming the blood clot that causes the heart attack. As long as the blood can squeeze by the narrowing caused by the cholesterol deposits in good volume, the heart will receive sufficient oxygen and nutrients to keep the heart tissue alive.

A critical factor then is to maintain the proper "slipperiness" of the blood cells and prevent a blood clot from forming in the coronary arteries. Pycnogenol® has a protective anti-aggregation (anti-clotting) effect on blood platelets. It is particularly effective against the damage to platelets from stress and smoking.

Pycnogenol's® mild hypotensive (blood pressure lowering) action helps maintain a normal blood pressure. Blood pressure is strongly influenced by nitric oxide levels in the blood, a compound that controls the relaxation of blood vessels and inhibits the angiotensin I converting enzyme (ACE), which raises blood pressure. Pycnogenol® maintains adequate nitric oxide levels, controlling vasorelaxation. (Fitzpatrick *et al.*, 1998) and inhibits angiotensin I converting enzyme (ACE), which promotes high blood pressure. (Blazso *et al.*, 1996)

Many recent studies have also linked inflammation to

heart disease. This inflammation, specifically of blood vessel walls, is likely related to the white blood cells drawn to oxidized LDL. Pycnogenol® reduces inflammation. (Blazso *et al.,* 1997)

Tears in the lining of arteries are another way in which deposits can form. Pycnogenol® is a factor in every way that vitamin E helps, as Pycnogenol® regenerates vitamin C, which in turn, regenerates vitamin E. (Cossins *et al.,* 1998) All of the antioxidants together form one terrific team to prevent heart disease.

Q. What are blood platelets and what do they do?

A. Blood platelets are small, disc-shaped, colorless blood cells. They are smaller than red blood cells and there are about 150,000 to 300,000 platelets per cubic centimeter of blood. It is uncanny to me, just how much a platelet looks like a chocolate chip cookie when observed through an electron microscope. Even granular proteins on the platelet surface resemble chocolate chips.

Platelets play a major role in the process of coagulation of blood to arrest bleeding (hemostasis). When bleeding begins, the vessel constricts, a protein called tissue factor is released and a protein (collagen) in the vessel wall is exposed. When tissue factor is released by the blood vessel wall, a lipoprotein on the surface of platelets called platelet factor 3 is activated and reacts with blood factors to promote the formation of a platelet plug and initiate other steps in the blood clotting mechanism. When platelet factor 3 is activated, the platelet changes shape and is said to be "activated."

However, platelets can be activated even when there is no bleeding, and this is not good. If they are activated they still tend to aggregate or clump together and initiate an undesirable blood clot which can block blood flow through the vessel and result in a heart attack or stroke. If this undesirable blood clot is stationary it is called a thrombus and if it travels through the vessel it is called an embolism. An embolism can reach a narrower vessel and become a thrombus.

Platelets can be activated by smoking, stress, in diabetes and certain nutritional deficiencies. As people age, a greater percentage of their platelets tend to be undesirably "activated."

Q. How does stress cause heart attacks?

A. When we are under stress, our adrenaline really flows. Adrenaline activates blood platelets to be prepared to clump together and form a blood clot. Furthermore, adrenaline causes blood vessels to constrict with the consequence of higher blood pressure. This was an advantage many years ago when we were attacked by wild animals. The blood platelets were prepared for an injury to more quickly form a blood clot and more efficiently prevent blood loss.

Nowadays, we live under permanent stress during the job, driving through traffic jams back home and never having enough time for anything. This causes permanent constriction of blood vessels as well as continuously "sticky" platelets.

In consequence the diameter of blood vessel is reduced leaving less space for the blood to flow. An atherosclerotic plaque may further reduce the space for blood flow. If now some platelets suddenly stick together and form a clot the vessel may be completely clogged and the surrounding tissue is no longer supplied with nutrients and oxygen. This is how heart infarction and stroke develop.

Q.   How does Pycnogenol® protect us from stress?

A.   Pycnogenol® can't make the cause of your stress go away. It improves the nitric oxide levels produced by cells lining the arteries. (Fitzpatrick *et al.,* 1998) The nitric oxide instructs muscles surrounding the blood vessels and causing them to relax. At the same time nitric oxide also instructs platelets to return back to their normal "non-sticky" condition, they no longer need to be "alarmed". Thus Pycnogenol® helps the body-own mechanism to counteract the activity of the stress hormone adrenaline. Pycnogenol® helps keep your blood "slippery" (as an anticoagulant) to reduce the chances of heart attacks and strokes.

Q.   How does Pycnogenol® help keep the blood slippery and free flowing to prevent the clots that cause heart attacks?

A.   Studies conducted by Dr. Peter Rohdewald in Germany and Dr. Ronald Watson in the United States show that Pycnogenol® blocks the effect of the stress hormone adrenaline on blood platelets, thereby reducing the platelets' tendency to clump together to form blood clots. When a person is under stress, large amounts of adrenaline are released, which cause the blood platelets to clump together. Pycnogenol® is particularly effective against increased platelet aggregation (stickiness and increased clotting tendency) caused by smoking. (Pütter *et al.,* 1999)

Dr. Watson's research (Araghi-Niknam et al., 1999) was published in *Cardiovascular Reviews Reports* in 1999 and was entitled "Reduction of Cardiovascular

Disease Risk Factors by French Maritime Pine Bark
Extract." A joint article by Drs. Watson, Rohdewald
and their colleagues was published in *Thrombosis
Research* in 1999 as "Inhibition of Smoking-Induced
Platelet Aggregation by Aspirin and Pycnogenol." (See
Pütter *et al*. 1999)

U. S. Patent # 5,720,956 was granted for Pycnogenol's®
ability to inhibit platelet aggregation.

Q. How much Pycnogenol® improve the blood of smokers?

A. In the clinical studies, the protective effect of a
single dose of 100 mg of Pycnogenol® was observed
within two hours and this protective effect lasted for
12 hours after ingestion, and a dose of 200 mg
protected the blood for up to two to three days . When
smokers took 200 milligrams of Pycnogenol® daily
for 60 days, their blood platelets return to almost
normal for non-smokers.

Q. How does Pycnogenol® restore sticky blood platelets to normal?

A. This protective effect of Pycnogenol® is achieved
by supporting the production of the body's-own
messenger molecule nitric oxide (somewhat like a
hormone). Nitric oxide is produced by cells forming
the inner lining of blood vessels. It acts on blood
platelets to "calm them down", to stop them being in a
state of alarm and "sticky", ready to form a blood clot.

Pycnogenol® inhibits platelet aggregation by inhibiting
the enzymes thromboxane A2, 5-lipoxygenase, and
other clotting compounds. Furthermore, this protection
comes without an increased risk of prolonged bleeding

times, or the side effects common to aspirin.

Furthermore, Pycnogenol® decreases the level of thromboxane, which is a vasoconstrictor (constricts blood vessels thereby reducing blood flow and increasing blood pressure) in smokers to the normal level for non-smokers. (Araghi-Niknam *et al.*, 1999)

Q. Isn't this the same way that aspirin works to prevent heart attacks?

A.   Not exactly, the difference, though technical, is important. Pycnogenol® supports the body's own production of nitric oxide, whereas aspirin irreversibly inhibits the enzyme cyclooxygenase.

Aspirin is widely prescribed by cardiologists to protect against heart attacks. The first studies showed that the proper dosage of aspirin can reduce the incidence of another heart attack in heart patients. Later studies showed that aspirin can also reduce the risk of having a first heart attack.

So far, this sounds good, but unfortunately, many people develop serious problems with prolonged aspirin use. They can develop ulcerated linings of the gastrointestinal tract and an increased tendency to bleed. Some people have been known to develop this condition suddenly and without warning. While aspirin therapy has benefit for many people, you should check with your doctor before taking it on a long-term basis.

On the other hand, Pycnogenol® is safe and does not cause increased bleeding or the side effects of aspirin. In the studies by Drs. Rohdewald and Watson, it was found that 100 milligrams of Pycnogenol® achieved the same desired effect on blood platelets in smokers as 500 mg of aspirin —and without the prolonged bleeding and other side effects of aspirin. (Pütter *et al.*, 1999)

Q. How does Pycnogenol® protect the linings of arteries?

A. Damage to the endothelium, or lining, of the heart and arteries contributes to the risk of heart disease. This damage can cause clots to form and allow cholesterol carriers to enter the artery walls. Researches at Loma Linda University, California, studied the protective effect of Pycnogenol® using arterial endothelial cells. They found that Pycnogenol® reduced the damage to endothelial cells caused by free radicals and through other noxious elements (Liu et al., 2000). They had earlier noted that Pycnogenol® increased production of other antioxidants in the cells (Wei *et al.,* 1997).

Q. How does Pycnogenol® relax blood vessels to help prevent high blood pressure?

A. Pycnogenol® does have a mild hypotensive (blood pressure lowering) effect that helps prevent high blood pressure. This effect is important, but it does not make Pycnogenol® an anti-hypertensive drug. There are two known reasons for this action. One mechanism involves the optimization of nitric oxide production in the blood vessels. Several researchers, including Dr. David Fitzpatrick of the University of South Florida and Dr. Lester Packer of the University of California, Berkeley, have conducted research on Pycnogenol® and nitric oxide, and how Pycnogenol® balances nitric oxide levels in the artery linings to facilitate blood flow. We will examine nitric oxide in more detail shortly.

A second mechanism involving angiotensin I converting enzyme (ACE) will be discussed shortly.

Q.   What is nitric oxide and why is it important?

A.   Nitric oxide has recently aroused much interest among scientists, though it was dismissed for decades as not being an important compound in the body— merely a waste product or inhaled air pollutant. Nitric oxide was named the "Molecule of the Year" in 1992 by the prestigious journal "Science." In 1998, three scientists were awarded Nobel Prizes for their research on nitric oxide. Now, we understand that it has far-reaching effects throughout the body.

Nitric oxide plays a role in many biochemical functions. It improves our memory and attention; it increases perfusion of kidneys, lungs and liver by enhancing blood flow; it preserves the functioning of the cardiovascular system; it is responsible for the male erection.

In terms of heart disease, readers may be familiar with the fact that during angina attacks (a pain in the heart due to insufficient blood flowing into the heart during exertion), patients find relief from taking nitroglycerin pills. These nitroglycerin pills release nitric oxide which relaxes the coronary arteries and allows more blood to flow into the heart.

Q.   How does Pycnogenol® optimize nitric oxide levels?

A.   The arteries inner lining, called the endothelium, produces nitric oxide which plays a role in the regulation of blood flow. In addition, the nitric oxide produced in the artery lining also acts to increase the production of a chemical messenger called cyclic-GMP (guanosine monophosphate), which is needed to keep blood platelets "slippery" and not prone to clumping or aggregation. Pycnogenol® stimulates the enzyme, nitric oxide synthase (NOS) to produce nitric oxide in the artery linings from the amino acid arginine.

Some nitric oxide is always needed, but too much can kill cells. Pycnogenol® helps regulate nitric oxide levels in the body at optimal levels. It helps the body produce adequate levels of nitric oxide for necessary functions, while reducing the levels of nitric oxide where it does harm.

Dr. David Fitzpatrick of the University of South Florida conducted tests to determine the effect of Pycnogenol® on portions of the aorta (the main artery from the heart). He found that it improved the production of nitric oxide in the endothelium, which in turn had a relaxing effect on the aorta in a dose-dependent manner. The results were published in 1998 in the *Journal of Cardiovascular Pharmacology* (Fitzpatrick *et al.*, 1998).

Q. Can Pycnogenol® also lower high blood pressure by blocking an enzyme that increases blood pressure?

A. Yes, Pycnogenol® blocks the action of angiotensin I converting enzyme (ACE) in causing high blood pressure. In this way, Pycnogenol® is similar to, but much safer than, common prescription drugs called "ACE inhibitors." ACE interferes with bradykinine, a compound that helps keep peripheral blood vessels properly dilated. Blocking this action leads towards a normalization of blood pressure without a danger of driving the blood pressure too low. It allows the bradykinine to act as it should, unencumbered by ACE.

Dr. Miklos Gabor and his colleagues at the Albert Szent-Györgyi Medical University in Szeged, Hungary, along with Dr. Peter Rohdewald of the University of Muenster, Germany found that Pycnogenol® has a dose-dependent action in blocking ACE from raising blood pressure. Based on their study, published in 1996 in *Pharmaceutical and Pharmacological Letters*, the researchers described the hypotensive effect of Pycnogenol® as "moderate" and people with normal or low blood pressure will not be affected, whereas those with high blood pressure due to too much ACE will benefit. The clinical study on this aspect is in progress at this writing in 2001 and the preliminary results are encouraging.

Q. Has any clinical study evaluated Pycnogenol® as an adjunct for treatment of high blood pressure.

A. A clinical study to be published by Dr. Ronald Watson of the University of Arizona in 2001 examined this possibility. Dr. Watson and his colleagues study is entitled "A randomized, double-blind, placebo-controlled, prospective, 16 week crossover study to determine the role of Pycnogenol® in modifying blood pressure in mildly hypertensive patients."

They found a significant decrease in the systolic blood pressure during Pycnogenol® supplementation. Also, serum thromboxane concentration was significantly decreased during Pycnogenol® supplementa-tion.(Araghi-Niknam *et al.*, 1999) The scientists concluded, "Our data suggest that supplementation with Pycnogenol® is effective in decreasing systolic blood pressure in hypertensive patients."

Q. **Can Pycnogenol® also reduce the inflammations that are now linked to heart disease?**

A. Yes, it can. Evidence shows that chronic inflammation from ordinary bacterial infections significantly increase the incidence of heart disease. It may seem strange to find that ordinary infections, such as periodontal (gum) disease, sinus infections, bronchitis, urinary tract infections and stomach ulcers, are linked to heart disease, but inflammation also activates white blood cells, which use free radicals to destroy bacteria and other "foreign" objects in the blood. These white blood cells migrate to the arteries where some of these free radicals leak out, oxidizing LDL and damaging the linings of arteries. The process also elevates a compound called C-reactive protein (CRP) in blood. Doctors are now considering elevated CRP levels as a risk factor in heart disease.

In a 2001 article in the American Heart Association's journal *Circulation*, it was reported that chronic infections may triple the risk of atherosclerosis, even when they don't have the classic risk factors such as high blood pressure, obesity, diabetes or lack of exercise.

Pycnogenol® helps in a couple of ways. As an antioxidant, it neutralizes these free radicals released by inflammation. Dr. Lau and his colleagues at Loma Linda University showed that it also decreases the body's production of cellular adhesion molecules (CAM), which help inflammatory cells to stick to blood vessel walls. (Peng *et al.*, 2000)

Q. How does Pycnogenol® improve blood circulation?

A. Pycnogenol® helps maintain good circulation in several ways. We have already discussed how Pycnogenol® improves blood flow via its effect on nitric oxide. Another way is that Pycnogenol® protects the endothelial cells that line the heart and blood vessels against free radicals. If they were damaged, the body would try to repair them, and this would result in scarring and lesions that reduce the flow of blood.

Pycnogenol® also binds to collagen and elastin, which are important proteins in blood vessels and skin. While bound to these proteins, Pycnogenol® blocks their degradation by certain enzymes. Pycnogenol® also facilitates the production of "ground substance," an intercellular cement that can fill much of the space between cells in the blood vessels and control the amount of fluid and compounds that can slip through. This also gives the blood vessels strength.

Q. Does Pycnogenol® improve the blood circulation in elderly people and how?

A. Yes. Dr. Watson has compared the tendency to form blood clots in a group of elderly people (average age 65) with a group of younger people (average age 32). He showed that the tendency of elderly people to form blood clots is significantly higher than in younger people. This is an explanation for the higher incidence of thrombus formation, heart infarction and stroke with higher age. After daily supplementation with Pycnogenol® over 8 weeks the tendency to form blood clots in the group of elderly people was almost normalized to the value found in the group of the 32 year olds. (Araghi-niknam, 1999) Pycnogenol® improves blood circulation in elderly through antithrombotic mechanism and by causing vaso-dilatation through optimal production of nitric oxide from endothelium as explained earlier.

Q. Is there a clinical study that examines several of these heart health benefits of Pycnogenol®?

A. A very interesting study was conducted in Beijing China and published in the *European Bulletin of Drug Research* in 1999. I had the opportunity to witness the first oral presentation of this study in Beijing in March 1999 and the second presentation in France in May 1999.

The study was led by Dr. Shiwen Wang of the Institute of Geriatric Cardiology at the PLA General Hospital in Beijing (Wang *et al.,* 1999) Sixty heart patients were studied for four weeks in a double-blind, placebo-controlled, randomized clinical trial. Blood microcirculation was measured by the diameter of the capillaries in the fingernail bed. Patients were monitored for adverse effects, electrocardiogram (ECG), myocardial ischemia and blood platelet aggregation, among other parameters.

Of the heart patients given 150 milligrams of Pycnogenol® three times a day for four weeks, 54% had improved microcirculation versus only 31% of those receiving a placebo (inert pill).

The study concluded, "Pycnogenol®" inhibited the adhesion and aggregation of platelets, enhanced the diameter of microvessels and microcirculation perfusion, and to some extent prevented and improved the myocardial ischemia in patients with coronary artery disease. There were no severe side effects nor toxicity to vital organs. Pycnogenol® can be used as a beneficial health protection agent to help preventing cardiovascular damage and thrombotic coronary artery disease. (Wang *et al.,* 1999)

CHAPTER 5

Pycnogenol Against Cancer and Degenerative Diseases

Pycnogenol® may have roles both as a preventive measure and as an adjunct to cancer therapy. It also has beneficial effects on the immune system, and is protective against degenerative diseases such as cancer, diabetes and arthritis. However, please do not interpret these findings as suggesting that Pycnogenol® is a "cure" for cancer.

"Cancer" is not a single disease, but actually a group of similar diseases. There are about 100 different types of cancer, and they all involve an abnormality of some of the body's cells. Cancers are merely cells growing wildly or uncontrolled. Most cancers involve tumors. The National Cancer Institute explains the production of tumors as follows:

"Healthy cells that make up the body's tissues grow, divide, and replace themselves in an orderly way. This process keeps the body in good repair. Sometimes, however, normal cells lose their ability to limit and direct their growth. They divide too rapidly and grow without order. Too much tissue is produced and tumors begin to be formed. Tumors can be either benign or malignant.

"Benign tumors are not cancerous. They do not spread to other parts of the body and they are seldom a threat to life. Often, benign tumors can be removed by surgery, and they are not likely to return.

"Malignant tumors are cancerous. They can invade and destroy nearby tissue and organs. Cancer cells also can spread, or metastasize, to other parts of the body, and form new tumors."

The key words are unregulated growth of cells. Free radicals can destroy or cause malfunction of the cells regulatory mechanism. Free radicals can cause cells to mutate and start the cancer process. How this is done will be discussed in the next question, but let us continue to look at the cancer development process for now.

The cancer development process is not the single-step of mutation alone. The major steps in cancer development include initiation, promotion, progression, cancer and metastasis. Just having a cell mutation will not necessarily lead to clinical cancer. The immune system can come into play and destroy mutated cells before they lead to cancer. The initiation process can involve gene alteration by DNA damage by free radicals, or it can involve the activation of an cancer gene called an oncogene. Chemicals called carcinogens can damage the DNA, but often these chemicals do not really harm DNA until they have been altered by a free radical

Let's examine how free radicals cause cancer.

1. Free radicals can damage DNA which causes the DNA to churn out the wrong stuff (material foreign to your body which is not really "you".) If the wrong stuff is produced, then the cell will die or be altered. An altered cell process is a mutation. Mutated cells can develop into cancer. Mutated cells can grow quickly because they are not sensed by neighboring cells as being normal tissue that should be regulated.

2. Free radicals can activate oncogenes of the DNA

that up-regulates the genetic expression of the so-called cancer genes.

3. Cells regulate their proliferation by their ability to sense the population of neighboring cells. Free radicals can damage cell membranes and inactivate the sensory mechanisms in the membrane that limit cell growth and reproduction. If a sensor becomes damaged, then cell proliferation and growth becomes uncontrolled.

4. Free radicals can activate carcinogens or pre-carcinogens to start the chemical reactions that lead to cancer.

5. Free radicals can suppress the immune system, inactivating the body's defense against cancer.

6. Antioxidants may have a role in apoptosis, which helps eliminate mutated cells from the body.

Even if several cells become mutated, cancer will not develop until these cells can reproduce more mutated cells and become associated in such a way as to develop their own blood supply and defense system. This step is called promotion. Some factors, such as alcohol, can speed this process. However, the immune system can still stop this stage until the cells develop their defenses against the body's immune system. Antioxidants can stop or slow each of the steps in cancer development. Preliminary evidence suggests that antioxidants can also reduce the chances of metastasis and boost the immune system. A very healthy immune system can even destroy full-blown clinical cancers.

Q.   How does Pycnogenol® help to protect against the very early development of cancer?

A.   Many epidemiological (population) studies have affirmed that diets rich in fruits and vegetables reduce the incidence of several cancers. Many scientists believe that the reason fruits and vegetables are so protective is that they are rich in antioxidants, especially vitamin C and bioflavonoids.

Pycnogenol® may help to protect against the very early causes of cancer in four ways: by destroying cancer-causing free radicals, by inactivating carcinogens, by preventing activation of oncogenes, by boosting your body's immune system so that any mutated cells can be destroyed before they become cancerous, and by reducing the tendency of cancer cells to stick together and adhere to other sites, in a process called metastasis. In addition, I believe that Pycnogenol® will also be found to inhibit several tumor promoters. This effect has been demonstrated with other bioflavonoids and explains part of their protective actions against cancers.

Free radicals damage the body's cell replicating system, which consists of deoxyribonucleic acid (DNA). DNA contains the templates to reproduce all of the cells in the body and is responsible for making you uniquely "You." If this template becomes damaged by free radicals, the body may not be able to repair all of the damage, and the result is that when the body does make a new cell, it may be a mutated cell, which can become benign (nonspreading) or malignant (cancerous) tumors.

Q. How can Pycnogenol® prevent cancer genes from being activated?

A. Reactive Oxygen Species (ROS) can activate genes

called oncogenes that can start the cancer process. ROS can cause a complex in cells called Nuclear Factor-kappa B (NF-kB) to dissociate and enter the cell nucleus where it binds to DNA and activates oncogenes.   Dr. Benjamin Lau (Loma Linda) and his colleagues have discovered that Pycnogenol® protects NF-kB from dissociation and from activating the oncogenes. (Peng *et al.,* 2000)

Q. Does Pycnogenol® directly protect DNA from the damage that can lead to cancer?

A.   Yes, Dr. Nelson and his colleagues have shown that Pycnogenol® can protect against hydroxyl radical-induced DNA damage. (Nelson *et al.,* 1998)

Q. Can Pycnogenol® deactivate carcinogens?

A.   Pycnogenol® inhibits the formation of reactive metabolites of the tobacco-specific nitrosamine (NNK), which has mutagenic and carcinogenic properties. (Huynh and Teel, 1998)

Q. How does Pycnogenol® boost immunity?

A.   In several ways. Dr. Ronald Watson of the University of Arizona, Tucson, specializes in studying the immune system and has conducted several studies with Pycnogenol® and the immune system. In one study, Dr. Watson found that Pycnogenol® boosted the levels of immune components called cytokines which play a crucial role in organizing the tactics of an immune response towards an infection. (Cheshier *et al.,* 1996)

Dr. Lau of the Loma Linda University showed that

Pycnogenol® can counteract the weakening power of the immune system by enhancing production of immune cells. This is especially important as a person ages and correlates well with the increasing risk for cancer with age.

All types of immune cells are important in the body's resistance to cancer. In an experiment by Dr. Watson, Pycnogenol® partially restored the decreased levels of certain cytokines in laboratory animals infected with a retrovirus very similar to HIV. In addition, Pycnogenol® greatly increased the activity of another type of immune cell, called natural killer cells, in infected mice. Pycnogenol® also strengthens immunity by protecting the existing immune components from their own chemicals. White blood cells use free radicals to destroy bacteria. When white blood cells over produce free radicals, white blood cells start to commit suicide. Pycnogenol® allows the bacteria to be killed while standing by to protect the white blood cells against any excess of free radicals.
(Cheshier *et al.*, 1996; Liu *et al.*, 1998; Peng *et al.*, 1999)

Q. Does boosting the immune system mean fewer colds and flus?

A. Most likely. The clinical trials haven't been carried out yet, but boosting your immune system means that you will have increased resistance to all of the diseases caused by germs. Dr. Lester Packer suggests[7] that, based on the study just discussed, Pycnogenol® should be able to shorten the duration of colds and flus. (see review article by Packer *et al.*, 1999)

Diabetes and Arthritis

Diabetes mellitus is a disorder in which the body cannot convert foods properly into energy. Arthritis is not one disease, but several diseases possibly having several causes. The word "arthritis" is derived from a Greek word meaning "joint" and actually means inflammation of the joint. As stressed often in this book, these diseases and many other degenerative diseases are either caused by or involve free radicals in their pathology

Q. What is so important about Pycnogenol® and diabetes?

A.   The damage to the cells that leads to either type 1 (juvenile) diabetes or type 2 (adult onset) diabetes may involve free radical reactions, but once the islets of Langerhans cells of the pancreas (type 1) or cellular mechanisms for utilizing insulin have been damaged, antioxidants can not reverse this. However, diabetes itself increases the production of free radicals, which further damage the body increasing the risk of heart attack, nerve damage (diabetic neuropathy), cataract (diabetic cataract), blindness (diabetic retinopathy) and more complications. Here's where powerful antioxidant protection is especially needed – diabetics need more antioxidant protection than healthy persons. Pycnogenol® is the most powerful antioxidant nutrient known at this time. Please see "diabtetic retinopathy" in Chapter 8 on "Eye Health."

Q. Does Pycnogenol® reduce inflammation?

A .   Yes. Inflammation is characterized by swelling, pain, localized heat, and redness. It can occur due to irritation or injury. Fluid gets trapped in the spaces between cells in the injured tissue. This fluid most often is the result of leakage from capillaries, but it can also be produced directly in tissue via free radical reactions. Inflammatory cells migrate into inflamed tissue and produce excessive amounts of free radicals. Pycnogenol® inhibits accumulation of inflammatory cells, and reduces the output of inflammatory substances. (Bayeta and Lau, 2001) Pycnogenol® helps normalize capillary permeability to prevent the leakage of fluid that causes edema (swelling). It also helps by neutralizing free radicals that promote swelling and inflammation. (Blazso *et al.,* 1994, 1995)

Q. So, can Pycnogenol® reduce the inflammation of arthritis?

A. When people with arthritis take Pycnogenol® for other disorders, they are often surprised to find that their arthritic aches and pains improve as well. This benefit should not be all that surprising because arthritis is an inflammatory disease that involves free radicals. Reducing free radicals eases the swelling associated with inflammation and improves the arthritic condition. A free radical called superoxide is involved in the inflammation of arthritis. This was demonstrated by the fact that injections of superoxide dismutase, an antioxidant that quenches the superoxide free radical, reduced the swelling and inflammation. Experiments by several investigators have shown that Pycnogenol® also quenches superoxide free radicals. (see review article by Packer *et al.*, 1999)

Q. Is Pycnogenol® effective against Lupus?

A. Systemic Lupus Erythematoses (SLE) is a multi-systemic autoimmune disease characterized by multiple immune dysfunction at the molecular and cellular level. It is considered a chronic inflammatory disease. Dr. S. Szegli and his Bucharest colleagues investigated Pycnogenol® in the treatment of SLE and concluded that "Pycnogenol®" was useful for second line therapy to reduce the inflammatory feature of SLE." (Stefanescu *et al.*, 2001)

CHAPTER 6

Effects on Aging, Athletic Performance, Healthy Lifestyle and Weight Control

Free radicals are involved in the aging process, and Pycnogenol® destroys free radicals, thus having an age-retarding effect. I will cite one study showing where Pycnogenol® extended the lifespan of a common laboratory species used to study the aging process, but there is more to aging than lifespan. The goal is to increase the quality of life as well as the length of life. We want to add more years to our lives, but we also want to add more life to our years. Slowing the aging process is all about living better and longer.

There is no one physical or mental condition directly attributed simply to the passage of time. It is not the passage of time that ages us, it is the accumulation of deleterious chemical events that deteriorates our body into the condition we call aged. Some of the alleged diseases or disorders associated with aging can also occur in the young. Children can have cancer, high blood pressure, arthritis and the like so it is not simply the number of years. What then is aging?

Aging is the process that reduces the number of healthy cells in the body. The most striking factor in the aging process is the body's loss of reserve due to the decreasing number of cells in each organ. For example, fasting blood glucose (blood sugar) levels remain fairly constant throughout life, but the glucose tolerance measurement shows a loss of response in aging. Glucose tolerance measures the reserve capacity of this system to respond to the stress of the glucose load used to challenge the system in the test. The same diminishment holds true for the recovery mechanisms of other systems. Simply stated the aging process is the body's loss of ability to respond to a challenge to its status quo (homeostasis). The mass of healthy active cells in each organ declines as a person ages, thus the organ's function is diminished.

Now the question becomes, what causes this loss of reserve? Free radical reactions result in the body's loss of active cells. The cumulative effect of billions of cellular free-radical reactions is the loss of cells. This happens in several ways.

1. Free radical damage to the cell membranes can impair the cell's ability to transport nutrients into the cell and the cell dies without replacing itself.

2. Free radical damage to cell membranes can impair the cell's ability to transport waste products out of the cell, thus the cell can strangle in its own waste. The result is that the cell can die without replacing itself.

3. Free radicals can damage the cell's DNA so that instead of the cell being replaced by another healthy daughter cell, the cell is replaced with a mutant that doesn't function correctly.

4. Free radicals can damage the lysosomal sac and release deadly lysosomes which are enzymes that destroy other cell components. This leaves the cell devoid of working parts and it can not be replaced. The cell becomes a clinker and the body becomes one cell older.

5. Free radicals can fuse proteins together in a fashion so as the proteins do not function properly. This can damage a cell so that it does not perform and does not reproduce a healthy replacement.

6. Free radical reactions form by-products such as the age pigment lipofuscin or advanced glycosolated end-products. These residues accumulate over time and interfere with cell function.

The result of many of the free radical reactions is that the number of active cells in the body decrease. This is analogous to the light bulbs on an old theater marquee that burn out one by one. For a while, the message can still be read, but as the number of burned-out bulbs increases, eventually the message is not discernible. In the body, the cells in each organ decline but the organ still functions until a point.

In addition to the many health benefits of Pycnogenol®, there are important "vanity" benefits as well. Pycnogenol® is often called the "skin vitamin" or the "oral cosmetic" because it rebuilds skin tissues, making it more flexible and smoother, which makes skin appear younger and healthier. It can't undo deep wrinkles or repair permanent sun damage, but it can make skin healthier and smoother.

Pycnogenol® can help improve the quality of life in many ways, as well as help reduce the risk of killer diseases and help us live *better* and longer.

Q. Have any lifespan or longevity studies been conducted with Pycnogenol®?

A. It is not practical to study humans in scientific lifespan studies because these studies would take too long and there are too many variables. Scientists find it more practical to study laboratory animals that have much shorter lifespan. Often, the studies begin with drosophila, a fruit fly, and then, if these studies are promising, laboratory rodents are studied.

Pycnogenol® lifespan studies are just beginning. Dr. L. Shuguang and his Chinese colleagues found that Pycnogenol® increased the average lifespan of drosophila by 13%. This would equate to an increase of nearly eight years for a person who otherwise would have a 70-year lifespan. It's a long way from fruit flies to humans, but at least the study shows that more studies are justified.

Pycnogenol® most likely increases lifespan by indirectly increasing cellular levels of superoxide dismutase and glutathione, as well as directly quenching free radicals throughout the body.

Q. Does Pycnogenol® help protect against Alzheimer's disease?

A. It's too early to tell, but laboratory studies are underway. We do know that Pycnogenol® shields brain cells from the oxidative stress of free radicals. One of the characteristics of Alzheimer's disease is the accumulation of the protein beta-amyloid. Dr. R. Schubert and his colleagues at the Salk Institute of Biological Sciences, San Diego, have found that Pycnogenol® prevents the toxic action of that protein against brain cells in laboratory experiments. (Liu *et al.,* 1998, 1999)

Dr. Lester Packer and colleagues at the University of California at Berkeley have found that Pycnogenol® protects brain cells from damage from excessive amounts of toxic glutamate. (Kobayashi *et al.,* 2000)

Q. Does Pycnogenol® improve memory or reduce the memory loss of aging?

A. Animal learning and memory studies are a good indication of what will apply to humans. Dr. Benjamin Lau and his colleagues at Loma Linda University in California investigated memory retention and learning ability of mice. They discovered that older mice given Pycnogenol® for two months almost retained the mental levels of young mice. (Liu, *et al.*, 1999)

Q. Does Pycnogenol® improve the beneficial effects of exercise?

A. Yes! I want to discuss the importance of Pycnogenol® in exercise and sports in this chapter. Exercise is beneficial in many ways, but few people realize that exercise increases the need for antioxidants. Sports and exercise require that we burn more calories for energy and consume more oxygen. When we consume more oxygen, we unfortunately create more free radicals. If we are deficient in antioxidants, the benefits of exercise are diminished by the damage from free radicals. The message here is not to reduce exercise or activity, but to be sure that you get adequate nourishment including ample antioxidants.

One study has even suggested that the powerful antioxidant Pycnogenol® improved athletic endurance. Since this is only one study involving a small number of people, it is not wise to extrapolate that study into a general recommendation. However, you should at least be informed of this study. Dr. Paul Pavlovic of the Department of Physical Education and Exercise Physiology at California State University found that in a double-blind, cross-over design clinical trail, the 24 persons receiving 200 milligrams of Pycnogenol®

daily for 30 days had an improvement in endurance of 21% over the time they did not take Pycnogenol® as measured by parameters such as maximal oxygen consumption. (Pavlovic, 1999)

Q. Does Pycnogenol® help people lose fat?

A. It may be helpful based on a few laboratory studies, but there is no evidence that merely taking Pycnogenol® supplements makes anyone slender. You will certainly find that lots of our, how should I say this, full-bodied friends, that take Pycnogenol® are healthier, but not necessarily slimmer. However, we can use any help that we can get, and it is encouraging that maybe a side benefit of taking Pycnogenol® is that it is working to reduce fat accumulation.

Dr. N. Hasegawa has published his research in *Phytotherapy Research* (14:472-473; 2000) showing that Pycnogenol® inhibits the accumulation of fat in fatty tissue. (Hasegawa, 2000). Dr. Hasegawa concludes that Pycnogenol® may contribute to the prevention of obesity. This study is a follow-up of his earlier study showing that Pycnogenol® stimulated the liberation of fat from fat cells (lipolysis). (*Phytotherapy Research* 13:619-620; 1999) It may indeed be that Pycnogenol® facilitates the expression (activation) of the genes that promote the breakdown of fat. The liberated fat may then become available to the cells for energy production. In any event, the question remains, "What happens to this fat that is broken down? Is it removed from the body? Does it become available energy? Does it return to the cells? More research is needed here.

CHAPTER 7

Effects on Varicose Veins, Edema, "Economy-Class Syndrome," Bruises and Venous Health

In addition to its protection against many diseases, Pycnogenol® also helps protect against varicose veins and bruises and helps reduce the severity of minor injuries. This protection is due to the bioflavonoids in Pycnogenol® and is not a general antioxidant effect. Pycnogenol® has been shown to improve venous health, help repair some varicose veins, and reduce the occurrence of new varicose veins. Fifteen clinical studies in venous disorders have been conducted with Pycnogenol® involving chronic venous insufficiency, varicose veins, thrombophlebitis, post-thrombotic syndrome and venous stasis edema. These studies have been reviewed by Dr. Om Gulati in the European Bulletin of Drug Research. (Gulati, 1999)

Q. How does Pycnogenol® strengthen veins and capillaries?

A. As I mentioned in the chapter on "Protecting the Heart and Circulation", one of the earliest discoveries about Pycnogenol® was its ability to strengthen capillaries, your body's tiniest blood vessels. Early research focused on the role of Pycnogenol® as either an independent factor or a co-factor with vitamin C in the maintenance of capillary health. Dr. Miklos Gabor of Albert Szent-Gyorgyi Medical University in Hungary conducted many studies over the years that demonstrate that Pycnogenol® improves capillary permeability and decreases capillary leakage and microbleeding.

Capillaries are not designed to be sealed against leakage. These blood vessels are the interface between the blood stream and oxygen, nutrients, and waste products. Capillaries must be permeable enough to allow fluids to seep out of the capillaries, mix with the fluid that surrounds all of the cells, and then reenter the capillaries. If the capillaries are too permeable, too much fluid and protein seep out, resulting in edema (swelling), and even red blood cells may seep out causing bruising and red spots (petechiae) or even hematomas.

Q. How is capillary permeability measured and studied?

A. Dr. Gabor measured the leakage of fluid through capillaries by using a device he invented called a petechiometer, which applies a vacuum over a small area of skin. The strength of the vacuum can be varied. The greater the vacuum required to produce petechiae, the higher the capillary strength of the permeability of the capillaries. Dr. Gabor and his colleagues have found that Pycnogenol® improved capillary strength within two hours and maintained it longer than eight hours. They have described their findings in the journal *Phlebologie in 1993.*

Q. Does Pycnogenol® protect against varicose veins and other symptoms of chronic venous insufficiency?

A. Dr. F. Feine-Haake, studied the benefit of 30 mg of Pycnogenol® given three times a day (a total of 90 mgs) on 100 persons having varicose veins and other symptoms of chronic venous insufficiency. Eighty percent showed a clear improvement, and 90 percent of them found that their nocturnal leg cramps also disappeared.

Pycnogenol® helps keep all of the blood vessels healthy and reduces edema in the legs, which contributes to the development of varicose veins. In double-blind, placebo-controlled studies it has been shown that Pycnogenol® greatly improves symptoms of chronic venous insufficiency. (Arcangeli, 2000; Petrassi *et al.,* 2000)

Q. Is Pycnogenol® effective against edema?

A. Clinical studies and laboratory animal studies show that Pycnogenol® reduces water retention and swelling in the legs due to edema, by strengthening capillaries and preventing leakage of fluids. (Gabor *et al* 1993; Blazso *et al.,* 1994; 1997; Arcangeli 2000; Petrassi *et al.,* 2000)

Q. How does Pycnogenol® prevent bruising and reduce the severity of minor injuries?

A. Pycnogenol® helps maintain capillary strength and proper capillary permeability. A bruise is pooled blood beneath the surface of the skin. If the capillaries leak too much, fluid and proteins can leak through the capillaries into the neighboring spaces between cells, thereby altering the normal osmotic pressure. Eventually, even red blood cells can leak through and spontaneously cause a bruise without a direct injury to the capillaries. Pycnogenol® restores proper permeability and reduces the incidence of spontaneous bruising. With stronger capillaries, it will take a more forceful injury to damage the veins and capillaries enough to allow microbleeding into the tissues.

Q. **If Pycnogenol® improves blood circulation and keeps blood flowing, would it be helpful for protection against swollen ankles and venous clots on long distance air flights – the so-called "Economy-Class Syndrome"?**

A. Medical experts and officials from 16 major airlines across the globe have gotten together under the auspices of the World Health Organization (March 11, 2001). Dr. John Scurr, a British vascular surgeon studied 200 people flying long distance. The results are to be published in the Lancet, a medical journal.

This is the only repeated question, so you can see how important I think it is. I wouldn't think of getting on a plane without taking extra Pycnogenol®. If my flight is longer than four hours, I take even more Pycnogenol® at the four-hour mark. I have seen too many people develop clots on flights, and more having embolisms lodging in their lungs a day or two after their flight as the clot dislodges from the leg vein and travels through the body.

The so-called "Economy Class Syndrome" is not limited to economy class flights. This condition has been blamed for at least 30 deaths in three years at just one hospital at London, England. Sitting still in airplane seats encourages the blood to pool in the ankles. The edge of the seat tends to reduce the return flow of the blood through the leg veins. One result is that the ankles can swell, but a worse result is that a blood clot can form in the deep veins of the legs and then travel as an embolism to a coronary artery and cause a heart attack or to the brain and cause a stroke. In addition, the reduced oxygen levels and increased radiation levels at high altitude flights increases the need for the powerful antioxidant protection of Pycnogenol®.

When you are trapped in a plane at high altitude, breathing germs from your neighbors for hours at a time, getting zapped by cosmic radiation, breathing low levels of oxygen, you definitely would benefit from extra Pycnogenol®. The first thing you will notice is that your shoes fit upon arrival. Airlines should be required to distribute Pycnogenol® supplements in flight just like they used to pass out chewing gum to help ease ear pressure changes.

Chapter 8

Eye Health

It's uncanny how many people have been introduced to the benefits of nutritional supplements because they have developed eye problems. There will be many more as the "baby boomers" age. Dry eyes, glaucoma and cataracts start to become a problem in the 50-plus years. Later on, age-related macular degeneration looms as a real danger.

The good news is that Pycnogenol® has been shown to improve visual acuity and suspend the deterioration of retinal function that can lead to blindness.

In addition, Pycnogenol® helps protect the eye lens against the free radicals generated by sunlight, and also reduces the risk of diabetic retinopathy. Also, Pycnogenol's® antioxidant power can help spare the dietary sparse vision-related nutrients, the carotenoids lutein and zeaxanthin, which protect the center of vision, the eye's macula.

One recent poll listed the possibility of lost vision as the number-two fear of senior citizens, second only to the fear of cancer. Pycnogenol® may be important to the body's defense against both.

Q. Has a clinical study really shown that Pycnogenol® can improve visual acuity?

A. Yes ! A double-blind, placebo-controlled study published in Phytotherapy in May, 2001 demonstrated that Pycnogenol® improved visual acuity in patients suffering from diabetes, atherosclerosis and other diseases. improved (Spadea and Balestrazzi, 2001)

The tests to measure eye health included the Snellen Chart (acuity at 20 feet) as well as visual field, opthalmoscopy, fluorangiography and electro-retinogram. Those receiving 50 milligrams of Pycnogenol®, three times a day had either an improvement in visual acuity or a slower rate of loss of acuity compared to those in the control group receiving a placebo (an inert pill) rather than Pycnogenol®.

Q.   Does Pycnogenol® protect against diabetic retinopathy?

A.   Five clinical studies conducted in Europe show that Pycnogenol® greatly improved symptoms in patients with diabetic retinopathies, maculopathies and other visual dysfunctions. The vision of treated patients not only stopped decreasing further, but even improved (Spadea and Balestrazzi, 2001) Pycnogenol® can improve these conditions because it not only protects the remaining healthy cells against free radical damage, Pycnogenol® also seals the microbleedings in the retina that obscures vision.

Q.   Has the protective effect of Pycnogenol® on the retina been studied in comparison to other antioxidants?

A.   Yes. In *in vitro* (test tube) studies, the potency of antioxidants to prevent damage of the very sensitive lipids of the eye retina, researchers in Japan found that Pycnogenol® was the most effective supplement, protecting these structure elements of the eye far better than grape seed extract or vitamin C and E (Chida *et* *al* 1999).

In these studies with retinal tissue, Pycnogenol® was 1.5 times more effective than catechin and at least ten times more potent than grape seed extract, 40 times more potent than vitamin E, 350 times more potent than vitamin C and 1,000 times more potent than lipoic acid.

In earlier *in vitro* studies, Pycnogenol® was found to be more effective in protecting the retina than several other antioxidants. (Ueda *et al.*, 1996)

Q.   Can Pycnogenol® help prevent cataracts?

A.   Cataracts are associated with aging, but they are caused by free radicals. Sunlight is the main source of free radicals that damage the eye lens. Several epidemiological studies have shown that various antioxidant nutrients reduce the incidence of cataracts. Since Pycnogenol® is water soluble, it can bathe the eye with its powerful combination of antioxidants.

A study by Dr. J. R. Trevithick of the University of Western Ontario in Canada has shown that Pycnogenol® helps to prevent cataract development in diabetic rats. (Trevithick *et al.,* 2000)

CHAPTER 9

Effects on Sexual Function, Fertility, PMS and Menstrual Disorders

By now it should be no surprise to learn that sexual function and dysfunction can be affected by free radicals. Perhaps this subject doesn't seem as important to many readers as the killer diseases, but for those suffering from infertility or other such disorders, this subject can be more important than the killers diseases.

Q. Can Pycnogenol® improve fertility?

A. Horse breeders swear by it, if that's any indication. It seems that antioxidants in general improve sperm motility and mobility. Especially useful is Pycnogenol®, but also vitamin C, selenium, lipoic acid, and vitamin E. Dr. Scott Roseff and colleagues at the West Essex Center for Advanced Reproductive Endocrinology in West Orange, New Jersey found that 200 milligrams of Pycnogenol® taken daily for 90 days increased the percentage of structurally normal sperm – that is – non-deformed sperm by an average of 99%. Sperm count did not change. They suggest that this 99-percent increase in structurally normal sperm may allow couples diagnosed with certain types of infertility to forgo *in vitro* fertilization in favor of less invasive and less expensive fertility-promoting procedures (Roseff and Gulati, 1999).

Q. Has the effect of Pycnogenol® been studied in menstrual cramps or other disorders and endometriosis?

A. Endometriosis is an abnormal condition in which the uterine mucous membrane invades other tissues in the pelvic cavity. Its typical symptoms include pelvic pain, pelvic mass, alteration of menses and infertility. Sometimes the pain can be incapacitating.

In a study by Drs. Takafumi Kohama and Nobutaka Suzuki of the School of Medicine of Kanazawa University, Japan, Pycnogenol® was given as a daily dose of 30-60 milligrams daily for four weeks, beginning two weeks before the period. The decrease or complete disappearance of pain occurred in 80% of the women with endometriosis, 70% of the women with severe menstrual pain and 60% of the women with post-operative gynecological surgery. (Kohama and Suzuki, 1999)

Pycnogenol® is spasmolytic (anti-spasmatic) and acts to reduce spasms of the uterus. The capillary protecting activity of Pycnogenol® may further contribute to soothe menstrual discomfort.

Q. Will Pycnogenol® help erectile dysfunction (impotence)?

A. In the chapter on Protecting the Heart and Circulation", we discussed nitric oxide and its most vital role in the male penile erection. It order for erection to occur, additional blood must flow into the penis. The arteries supplying this blood depend on nitric oxide to allow them to relax and permit additional blood flow. This nitric oxide is made in the lining of the arteries by the enzyme nitric oxide synthase using the amino acid arginine. Pycnogenol® can stimulate the production of this enzyme and thus increase the production of the needed nitric oxide.

The drug Viagra also works through a mechanism that increases nitric oxide production in these arteries. Studies are planned to determine if Pycnogenol® will be effective, as the theory and many reports suggests. Persons who can't wait for the study results, may want to try supplementing their diet with both Pycnogenol® and l-arginine for several weeks.

CHAPTER 10

Effects on Allergies

The exciting news about the many roles of Pycnogenol® in reducing the risk of the killer diseases, such as cancer and heart disease, has been uncovered fairly recently as researchers studied its antioxidant functions. However, decades before Pycnogenol's® antioxidant roles were known, it was successfully used – especially in Europe — to control hay fever and other allergies. It has also been known for decades that Pycnogenol® fights inflammation, although the reason wasn't clear until recently.

Q. What are allergies?

A. Allergies are hypersensitive reactions that occur when the body comes in contact with harmless substances that the body perceives as harmful. Substances that cause these reactions are termed allergens. When a hypersensitive person comes into contact with an allergen, the body releases histamine in an attempt to fight off the allergen. This release of histamine triggers the symptoms so common to allergies—inflammation, sneezing, runny nose, and itchy eyes.

Q. How does Pycnogenol® ease the symptoms of allergies?

A. Bioflavonoids appears to block histamine release in *in vitro* studies. Professor Sharma from the Department of Pharmacology of the University of Dublin has shown that Pycnogenol® inhibits histamine release from specific body cells (mast cells). This action is mediated through free-radical scavenging property of Pycnogenol®. These findings were presented during the British Pharmacology Society meetings held in Dublin in July 2001. (Sharma, 2001)

Antihistamines generally work by interfering with the attachment of histamine to cells after its been released. It's more efficient to prevent histamine release in the first place than to try to keep released histamine away from its receptors on target cells.

Bioflavonoids also appears to increase the uptake and re-uptake of histamine into its storage granules, where it's out of the way and can't cause misery.

Pycnogenol® may be effective against allergies without producing side effects as drowsiness and dry mucous membranes.

CHAPTER 11

Attention Deficit
Hyperactivity Disorder (ADHD)

Attention deficit disorder (ADD) and attention deficit hyperactivity disorder (ADHD) are a group of behavioral problems that used to be called hyperactivity. They involve impulsive behavior, the inability to keep focused on a task, and/or hyperactivity. I learned quite unexpectedly that Pycnogenol® may be helpful in the treatment of these disorders as well.

Q. How many people are affected by ADD and ADHD, and are they all children ?

A. ADD and ADHD affect about 5 to 7 percent of the population. ADD and ADHD affects males about ten times more often than females. These conditions normally begin by four to seven years of age and seem to peak between eight and ten years of age. However, adolescents and adults also suffer from ADD and ADHD. From 30 to 70 percent of affected children are left untreated and grow to become adults with these disorders. ADD and ADHD rarely manifest themselves as adult-onset disorders. The physical hyperactivity lessens with age, but the adult still has marked attention problems and can be impulsive. Problems in the adolescent and adult occur predominantly as academic failure, low self-esteem, and difficulty learning appropriate social behavior. Often, those with ADD and ADHD have personality-trait disorders, antisocial behavior, short attention spans, and poor social skills, and are impulsive and restless.

Q. What is the cause of ADD?

A. The cause of ADD and ADHD is not known, but structural abnormalities have been ruled out. The leading suspect appears to be problems with neurotransmitters, possibly associated with decreased activity or stimulation in the upper brainstem and frontal midbrain. There is also suspicion that toxins, environmental problems, or neurological immaturity could be causative factors.

Q. All kids seem a little hyperactive at one time or another. What are the official symptoms of ADD?

A. The American Psychiatric Association lists fourteen signs, of which at least eight must be present to be officially classified as ADD. These fourteen signs are:

1. Often fidgeting with hands or feet, or squirming while seated.

2. Having difficulty remaining seated when required to do so.

3. Being easily distracted by extraneous stimuli.

4. Having difficulty awaiting turn in games or group activities.

5. Often blurting out answers before questions are

completed.

6. Having difficulty in following instructions.

7. Having difficulty sustaining attention in tasks or play activities.

8. Often shifting from one uncompleted task to another.

9. Having difficulty playing quietly.

10. Often talking excessively.

11. Often interrupting or intruding on others.

12. Often not listening to what is being said.

13. Often forgetting things necessary for tasks or activities.

14. Often engaging in physically dangerous activities without considering possible consequences.

Q. What is the conventional treatment for ADD?

A. The conventional treatment is with central nervous system stimulants, such as amphetamines. Stimulants seem to have a calming effect on children. Ritalin (methylphenidate hydrochloride) is widely prescribed, and some people have estimated that 5 to 10 percent of our youngsters go to school on this prescription drug. According to the Merck Manual, common side effects of Ritalin are sleep disturbances, depression, headache, stomach ache, suppressed appetite, elevated blood pressure, decreased learning, behavioral changes, and reduction of growth.

Q. How could Pycnogenol® help those with ADD?

A. One way is that the antioxidant effect of Pycnogenol® keeps neurotransmitters functioning longer. Pycnogenol® also improves circulation, including microcirculation in the brain. The increased production of nitric oxide, which also acts as neurotransmitter, may contribute to the improvement of memory and learning ability. However, I suspect that the effect of Pycnogenol® is more complex than this. It will take more research to uncover exactly how Pycnogenol® functions to help those with ADD and to improve cognitive function in general.

Q. How was the apparent benefit of Pycnogenol® to those with ADD discovered?

A. I'll take credit for being the first to report this apparent benefit at a scientific meeting, but the discovery has been made unexpectedly by many individuals. A common example is that persons taking Pycnogenol® for their hay fever found that their ADD symptoms decreased in a week or two. Through the years, because I was the author of two other books on Pycnogenol®, I have received hundreds of letters reporting this.

I surveyed the case histories and recent experience of several patients and found that Pycnogenol® had helped all of the patients who tried it. I reported this small study at The Second International Pycnogenol® Symposium in May 1995 in Biarritz, France.

In August 1995, 1 received a letter from psychologist Julie Paul, Ph.D., who confirmed that Pycnogenol® had also helped her immensely, as well as her colleague, Dr. Stephen Tennenbaum.

**Q.   Have any studies of Pycnogenol® and ADD
been reported in the medical literature?**

A.   There are case reports in the medical literature,
but I am not aware of any large clinical trials at this
writing. One case report was described in the *Journal
of the American Academy of Child & Adolescent
Psychiatry* (38:4; 357-358; 1999) by Dr. Steven
Heimann of Evansville Indiana.

Dr. Heimann tells of a child not responding well to
drug therapy, but responding well to Pycnogenol®
given to him by his parents. Dr. Heimann studied the
effects of Pycnogenol® by taking the child off
Pycnogenol® and then re-introducing it. As Dr.
Heimann reports, "The parents reluctantly agreed to
give the child a trial off Pycnogenol® for four weeks
to compare the effects of (drug) plus Pycnogenol® to
(drug) alone. Within two weeks of stopping
Pycnogenol® the patient became significantly more
hyperactive and impulsive, marked by numerous
demerits in school. He was also involved in several
physical altercations, which previously had abated with
Pycnogenol®. The child's regimen of Pycnogenol® was
reinstated, and again he demonstrated significant
improvement in ADHD target symptoms within three
weeks."

In Japan, Dr. Hayashi Masao, a neurologist in Kani-
city, Gifu Prefecture reported that Pycnogenol® had
therapeutic effect in the treatment of ADHD symptoms
in children. He concludes, "Although we still need
more evidence of the effect of Pycnogenol® in the
treatment of ADHD, it is time to carry out the clinical
trials to prove it."

Also, Dr. Jesse Lynn Hanley describes in her book
"Attention deficit disorder" that Pycnogenol® would
be a staple in her treatment of people with ADD
symptoms. (Hanley, H., 2000)

Still, it is too early to make a claim that Pycnogenol®
has been shown scientifically to improve ADD
symptoms. However, I have seen enough preliminary
anecdotal evidence to be personally convinced that the
full scientific proof will be forthcoming.

Chapter 12

Skincare and Cosmetics

Pycnogenol® has been called "the skin vitamin" by many users. However, as explained earlier, Pycnogenol® is not a vitamin, but a nutritional supplement. It has also been popularly called "the oral cosmetic" because it rebuilds skin tissues, making skin more flexible and smoother which makes skin appear younger and healthier. Pycnogenol® can't undo deep wrinkles or repair the permanent sun damage of actinic kerotosis, but it can make skin healthier, livelier, and smoother.

Pycnogenol's® first commercial uses were based on its ability to improve the permeability of blood capillaries by improving the production of "ground substance" between the cells. This was part of the explanation as to why Pycnogenol®-like decoction used by the North American Indians cured scurvy. Soon it was also learned that Pycnogenol® improves skin by promoting and protecting the skin proteins, collagen and elastin.

Q. How does Pycnogenol® contribute to skin smoothness?

A. In addition to its protective benefits against free radicals, which prevents skin damage, Pycnogenol® binds to collagen and elastin, two major skin proteins, and protects it from various enzymes that break it down. This action reduces the thinning of skin that develops with aging. Pycnogenol® helps the skin rebuild its thickness and elasticity. Skin fullness and elasticity are essential for skin smoothness.

Q.   How does Pycnogenol® make skin younger looking?

A.   As skin ages, it loses its flexibility. This is primarily due to the cumulative effect of sun exposure, which alters the skin structure and reduces the amount of skin protein produced. You can easily see this effect. When young skin is pinched and pulled up, it will spring back quickly. When older skin is similarly pinched, it returns to position very slowly. Try this on the back of the hands of people of various ages. How does your skin do?

Have you ever noticed that the skin on the back of the necks of farmers and fishermen is thick, leathery, and deeply wrinkled compared to the skin of office workers? You can also compare the apparent age of skin on different areas of your own body. We tend to think of the skin of our bodies as being the same age as our chronological age, but the fact is that some cells are much newer than others.

Compare the smoothness of the skin on a sun-exposed area, such as the back of your neck, to the skin on a sun-protected area, such as your buttocks. The sun is what made the difference, by causing free radicals that fused molecules of the skin protein collagen together.

The proteins in young skin freely slide over each other and spring back to their normal length when stretched. As time goes by and exposure to the sun accumulates, the ultraviolet energy in sunlight interacts with fats in the skin to produce free radicals. These free radicals damage proteins in the skin and can link the proteins together. These damaged proteins do not easily slide over one another and do not recoil rapidly. How does Pycnogenol® fit in? By neutralizing free radicals, Pycnogenol® can lessen sun damage to skin.

Q. Can Pycnogenol® help protect from sunburn as well as the long-term damage that ages skin?

A.   To some extent it can. People who are well protected by antioxidants, such as Pycnogenol®, find that their skin does not "burn" as quickly in the sun. Sunburn is an inflammation resulting from the free-radicals produced by the effect of sunlight on fats in the skin. Free-radical damage can be limited by the scavenging effect of the antioxidants. Studies have shown that the time of exposure required for sunburn to develop can be increased with Pycnogenol®, but Pycnogenol® should not be your only protection from the sun. The use of sunblock, wearing a hat, and an awareness of exposure time are also important.

Q. Can Pycnogenol® be used as an external sunscreen as well as an internal sunscreen?

A.   Yes, it can. In experiments, Dr. Peter Rohdewald of the University of Munster in Germany, marked different areas of the forearm, applied different strengths of Pycnogenol® to these areas, then exposed the forearm to sunlight. Pycnogenol® protected the skin in a dose-related manner, meaning that higher concentrations were better than lower concentrations. Several other researchers have extended these studies and shown that human volunteers were more resistant to UV irradiation when they had taken Pycnogenol®

tablets (Saliou *et al.*, 2001). They also discovered that Pycnogenol® prevents inflammation of the UV-exposed skin.

Q.   Can Pycnogenol® cure psoriasis?

A.   Psoriasis is characterized by capillary bleeding associated with increased capillary fragility. The capillary resistance of psoriatic patients is significantly lower than that of healthy persons. According to Dr. Miklos Gabor of the Albert Szent-Gyorgyi Medical University, Hungary, Pycnogenol® helps improve capillary resistance.

Although there are no clinical studies to verify this action, holistic physicians in Europe and in the United States have experienced good effects with Pycnogenol® in psoriasis. Many have unexpectedly found that when Pycnogenol® was given to patients for other disorders, the patients' psoriasis suddenly cleared up. A recent study by Dr. Packer has revealed how Pycnogenol® can be effective against psoriasis and other skin disorders: It acts on genes encoding inflammatory molecules. Pycnogenol® reduces production of these molecules, and thus turns off the inflammation. (Rihn *et al.,* 2001)

Q.   Is Pycnogenol® useful in cases of skin hyper-pigmentation?

A.   Melasma (chloasma) is a disorder of cutaneous hyperpigmentation affecting the sun-exposed area of the skin such as faces mainly of women. Dr. Ni Zhigang and his colleagues at the Chinese Academy of Traditional Chinese Medicine found that 30 days of treatment with 75 milligrams of Pycnogenol® daily to be very effective and safe. Eighty percent of patients responded very favorably with the area of hyperpigmentation and the intensity of hyperpigmentation greatly reduced.

CHAPTER 13
How to Use Pycnogenol®

If you now believe, as I do, that Pycnogenol® may help you, you'll probably want some information on how to take it. This final chapter answers these practical, everyday questions. Select a brand that you trust, determine the concentration suited for your purposes, and double-check to see if the label carries the Pycnogenol® trademark (logo of pine tree) or patent number, or mentions that it was produced by Horphag Research. If none of these notations appear on the label, you have an imitation, not Pycnogenol®.

Q.   How much Pycnogenol® do I need?

A.   This depends on why you wish to take Pycnogenol®. If you just want to improve the synergistic effect of your nutritional antioxidants, you need only 20 to 25 mg of Pycnogenol® a day. If you are seeking to optimize your antioxidant defenses, you may wish to take 50 to 100 mg a day. If you wish to protect your blood platelets from stress or smoke, or reduce pain or swelling, due to venous disorder or diabetic retinopathy then you may need to take one-half to one mg for every pound of your body weight. As the condition improves, you may be able to start cutting this back to the 50 to 100 mg per day range.

Q. Is it better to take Pycnogenol® on an empty stomach or with meals?

A. Taking Pycnogenol® with meals or on an empty stomach does not affect absorption, and Pycnogenol® does not produce any digestive disturbances, so it really doesn't matter when you take it. However, most people find that taking supplements with meals is easier, more convenient, and gentler on the system. Bioflavonoids, such as Pycnogenol®, improve the absorption of vitamin C, so it is wise to take Pycnogenol® with your other supplements, and it is probably more convenient to take Pycnogenol® at the same time you take your other supplements and with meals.

Q. Is it better to take Pycnogenol® in the morning or at night?

A. As with vitamin C and other water-soluble nutrients, Pycnogenol® is most effective when taken in divided dosages spread out over two or three times a day. This maintains a constant level of Pycnogenol® in the blood. However, there is no reason that your daily amount of Pycnogenol® cannot be taken all at once. However, people from Asia reported that they were too active and could not sleep when they had the full dose of Pycnogenol® in the evening.

Q. Who should take Pycnogenol®?

A. There are no known contraindications-conditions under which Pycnogenol® should not be used. As always, pregnant women and small children should consult with their health care practitioner before taking any dietary supplement, herb or medication. If your doctor has prescribed anticoagulants you should ask him whether you may also use Pycnogenol®, as it will also decrease the reactivity of blood platelets. The doctor may choose to lower the drug dosage.

Q. Is Pycnogenol® safe to take?

A. Yes, it is. Millions of users regularly take Pycnogenol® as a dietary supplement and to improve many health conditions. Pycnogenol® has been in wide usage since the late 1960s with no reported serious adverse health effects. It has been studied by toxicologists who have concluded that Pycnogenol® is safe.

Dozens and dozens of studies through the many years of use have shown that Pycnogenol® is nontoxic, non-mutagenic (doesn't cause mutations in DNA), and noncarcinogenic (doesn't cause cancer). Studies also indicate that Pycnogenol® will not cause birth defects, but I would never suggest that a woman start taking any supplement without first checking with her physician.

Dr. Peter Rohdewald has overseen safety studies of Pycnogenol® since 1982. He is a pharmaceutical researcher and teaches pharmaceutical science. He is well versed in toxicology and the safety of nutrients and drugs and has served as the Commissarial Director of the Institute for Pharmaceutical Chemistry at the University of Muenster.

Several acute toxicity studies found that it would take 336 grams-nearly one pound-to cause any type of toxic effects in a 155-pound person. Studies of long-term toxicity found that adverse effects would not be produced until 11250 milligrams a day were taken for more than six months by a 150-pound person. The highest recommended dose of Pycnogenol® is about 360 milligrams a day in studies on venous disorders.

There were no side effects. More typical dosages would be in the 50 to 100 milligrams per day range. Pycnogenol® is safe as a daily food supplement when taken as recommended.

CHAPTER 14

Conclusion

By now, you understand why Pycnogenol® has excited so many people. It can help protect you from a variety of diseases—including various types of heart disease and circulatory disorders—aggravated by free radicals. It can boost your immune system and also help protect you from infectious diseases.

As scientists have become excited about Pycnogenol®, it has motivated them to investigate and discover the specific and highly detailed mechanisms of how it works. They are learning about how Pycnogenol® interacts with nitric oxide, cellular adhesion molecules, and many other biochemical molecules.

Such details may not be of interest to you. Odds are that the health benefits of Pycnogenol® are of much greater interest. In writing about Pycnogenol® and in frequently talking with scientists doing the actual research on this remarkable substance, I have continued to be impressed by its positive effects on health. Obviously, I take it myself, and, perhaps not surprisingly, I think that everyone could benefit from Pycnogenol® supplements.

GLOSSARY

Aggregation. Assembling, clumping, or sticking together.

Antioxidant. Compounds that protect other compounds against oxidation and free radicals.

Bioavailability. The rate at which a nutrient is made available for action in the body.

Bioflavonoids. A family of beneficial compounds with a crystalline structure, which are found in plants.

Collagen. A protein that composes much of connective tissue and skin.

Enzymes. Proteins that initiate specific reactions in the body.

Free radical. An atom or molecule with at least one unpaired electron that damages body components and can lead to many diseases.

Oxidation. The reaction of a compound with oxygen, or a reaction in which an atom loses an electron.

Platelets. Small blood cells involved in forming blood clots.

Proanthocyanidins. Another name for procyanidins.

100

Procyanidins. A subclass of bioflavonoids to which Pycnogenol® belongs.

Pycnogenol®. A nutritional supplement, composed of bioflavonoids and organic acids, that has several beneficial effects in the body, including antioxidant activities, immune boosting effects, and cardiovascular protective properties.

BIBLIOGRAPY

Araghi-Nicknam, M., Hosseini, S., Larson D., Rohdewald, P. and Watson R.R. (1999)
Pine bark extract reduces platelet aggregation.
Integrative Medicine, 2 (2/3): 73-77.

Arcangeli, P. (2000)
Pycnogenol® in chronic venous insufficiency.
Fitoterapia, 71: 236-244.

Bayeta, E. and Lau, B.H.S. (1999)
Pycnogenol® inhibits generation of inflammatory mediators in the macrophages
Nutrition Res., 20: 249-259.

Blazso, G., Gabor, M., Sibbel, R. and Rohdewald, P. (1994)
Anti-inflammatory and superoxide radical scavenging activities of procyanidins containing extract from the bark of *Pinus pinaster* sol. and its fractions.
Pharm. Parmacol. Lett., 3: 217-220.

Blazso, G., Rohdewald, P., Sibbel, R. and Gabor, M. (1995)
Anti-inflammatory activities of procyanidin-containing extracts from Pinus pinaster sol.
Proceedings of the International Bioflavonoid Symposium, Vienna, Austria, ed. Antus, S., Gabor, M. and Vetschera, K. July 16-19, 1995, pages 231-238.

Blazso, G., Gaspar R., Gabor, M., Rüve H-J and Rohdewald, P. (1996)
ACE inhibition and hypotensive effect of procyanidins containing extract from the bark of *Pinus pinaster* Sol.
Pharm. Pharmacol. Lett., 6 (1): 8-11.

Blazso, G., Gabor, M. and Rohdewald, P. (1997)
Antiinflammatory activities of procyanidin containing extracts *from Pinus pinaster* Ait. after oral and cutaneous application.
Pharmazie, 52 (5): 380-382.

102

Cheshier, J.E., Ardestani-Kaboudanian, S., Liang B., Araghi-nicknam, M., Chung, S., Lane, L., Castro, A. and Watson, R.R. (1996)
Immuno-modulation by Pycnogenol® in retro-virus infected or ethanol-fed mice.
Life Sci., 58(5): 87-96.

Chida, M., Suzuki, K., Nakanishi-Ueda, T., Ueda, T., Yasuhara, H., Koide, R. and Armstrong, D. (1999)
In vitro testing of antioxidants and biochemical end-points in bovine retinal tissue.
Ophthalmic Research, 31: 407-415.

Cossins, E., Lee, R. and Packer, L. (1998)
ESR studies of vitamin C regeneration, order of reaetivity of natural source phytochemical preparations.
Biochem Mol. Biol. Int., 45 (3): 583-597.

Drehsen, G. (1999)
From ancient pine bark uses to Pycnogenol®, *In "Antioxidant Food Supplements in human health", ed. L. Packer, M. Hiramatsu and T. Yoshikawa, published by Academic Press, 1999, Chapter 20, pages 311-322.*

Fitzpatrick, D.F., Bing, B. and Rohdewald, P. (1998)
Endothelium-dependent vascular effects of Pycnogenol®.
Journal Cardiovascular Pharmacology, 32: 509-515.

Gabor, M., Engi, E. and Sonkodi, S. (1993)
Die Kapillarwandresistenz und ihre Beeinflussung durch wasserlösliche Flavonderivate bei spontan hypertonischen Ratten.
Phlebologie, 22: 178-182.

Gulati, O. P. (1999)
Pycnogenol® in venous disorders: A review.
European Bulletin of Drug Research, 7 (2): 8-13.

Guochang, Z. (1993)
Ultraviolet radiation-induced oxidative stress in cultured human skin fibroblasts and antioxidant protection.
Ph.D. Thesis, University of Jyväskylä, 33: 1-86, Jyväskylä, Finland.

Hasegawa, N. (1999)
Stimulation of lipolysis by Pycnogenol®.
Phytotherapy Research, 13: 619-620.

Hasegawa, N. (2000)
Inhibition of lipogenesis by Pycnogenol®.
Phytotherapy Research, 14: 472-473.

Huynh, H.T. and Teel, R.W. (1998)
Effects of Pycnogenol® on the microsomal metabolism of the tobacco-specific nitrosamine NNK as a function of age.
Cancer letters, 132: 135-139.

Huynh, H.T. and Teel R.W. (2000)
Selective induction of apoptosis in human mammary cancer cells (MCF-7) by Pycnogenol®.
Anticancer Research, 20 (4): 2417-2420.

Kobayashi, M.S., Han, D., and Packer, L. (2000)
Antioxidants and herbal extracts protect HT-4 neuronal cells against glutamate-induced cytotoxicity
Free Rad. Res., 32: 115-124.

Kohama, T. and Suzuki, N. (1999)
The treatment of gynaecological disorders with Pycnogenol®.
European Bulletin of Drug Research, 7 (2):30-32.

Liu, F.J., Zhang, Y.X. and Lau B.H.S. (1998)
Pycnogenol® enhances immune and haemopoietic function in senescence-accelerated mice.
CMLS, Cell. Mol. Life. Sci., 54: 1168-1172.

Liu, F., Zhang, Y., and Lau, B.H.S. (1999)
Pycnogenol® improves learning impairment and memory deficit in senescence-accelerated mice.
Journal of Anti-aging Medicine, 2 (4): 349-355.

Liu, F. Lau, B.H.S., Peng, Q and Shah, V. (2000)
Pycnogenol® protects vascular endothelial cells from b-amyloid-induced injury.
Biol. Pharm. Bull, 23 (6): 735-737.

Nelson, A.B., Lau, B.H.S., Ide, N. and Rong, Y. (1998)
Pycnogenol® inhibits macrophage oxidative burst, lipoprotein oxidation and hydroxyl radical-induced DNA damage.
Drug Development and Industrial Pharmacy, 24 (2): 139-144.

Noda, Y., Anzai, K., Mori, A., Kohno, M., Shinmei, M. and Packer, L. (1997)
Hydroxyl and superoxide anion radical scavenging activities of natural source antioxidants using the computerized JES-FR30 ESR spectrometer system.
Biochem. & Mol. Biol. Int., 42 (1): 35-44.

Packer, L., Rimbach, G. and Virgili, F. (1999)
Antioxidant activity and biologic properties of a procyanidin-rich extract from the pine (Pinus maritima) bark, Pycnogenol®.
Review Article In Free Radical Biology and Medicine, 27(5/6): 704-724.

Pavlovic, P. (1999)
Improved endurance by use of antioxidants.
European Bulletin of Drug Research, 7 (2): 26-29.

Peng, Q., Wei, Z. and Lau B.H.S. (2000)
Pycnogenol® inhibits tumor necrosis factor-a(TNF-a)-induced nuclear factor kappa B activation, and adhesion molecule expression in human vascular endothelial cells.
CMLS. Cell. Mol. Life Sci., 57: 834-841.

Petrassi, C., Mastromarino, A. and Spartera, C. (2000).
Pycnogenol® in chronic venous insufficiency.
Phytomedicine 7(5): 383-388.

Pütter, M., Grotemeyer, K.H.M., Würthwein, G., Araghi-Nicknam, M., Watson R.R., Hosseini, S. and Rohdewald, P. (1999)
Inhibition of smoking-induced platelet aggregation by aspirin and Pycnogenol®.
Thrombosis Research, 95: 155-161.

Rihn, B., Saliou, C., Bottin, M.C., Keith, G. and Packer, L. (2001)
From ancient remedies to modern therapeutics: Pine bark uses in skin disorders revisited,
Phytotherapie Research, 15: 76-78.

Rong Y., Li, L., Shah, V. and Lau, B.H.S. (1995)
Pycnogenol® protects vascular endothelial cells from t-butyl hydroperoxide induced oxidant injury.
Biotechnology Therapeutics, 5 (3 & 4): 117-126.

Roseff, S and Gulati, R. (1999)
Improvement of sperm quality by Pycnogenol®.
European Bulletin of Drug Research, 7 (2): 33-36.

Saliou, C., Rimbach, G., Moini, H., McLaughlin, L., Hosseini, S., Lee, J., Watson, R.R., Packer, L. (2001)
Solar ultraviolet-induced erythema in human skin and nuclear factor-kappa-B-dependent gene expression in keratinocytes are modilated by a French maritime pine bark extract.
Free Radical Biology and Medicine, 30(2): 154-160.

Sharma, S. C.
Effect of Pycnogenol® on Mast Cell Histamine Release.
Proc. Brit. Pharmacol. Soc., July 3-5 2001 p44)

Spadea, L., Balestrazzi, E. (2001)
Treatment of vascular retinopathies with Pycnogenol®.
Phytotherapie Research **15**:*1-5 .*

Stefanescu, M., Matache, C., Onu, A., Tanaseanu, S., Dragomir, C.,
Constantinescu, I., Schönlau, F., Rohdewald, P and Szegli, G. (2001)
Pycnogenol®'s efficacy in the treatment of systemic lupus erythematosus patients.
Phytotherapie Research (in press)

Trevithick *et al.*, 2000
Pycnogenol®, antioxidant, and cataract risk reduction experiments.
Investigative Ophthamology & Visual Sci. **41(4)** Suppl S 1101 B476 (Mar 15 2000)

Ueda, T., Ueda, T. and Armstrong, D. (1996)
Preventive effects of natural and synthetic antioxidants on lipid peroxidation in the mammalian eye.
Ophthalmic Res. *28: 184-192.*

Virgili F., Kim, D. and Packer, L. (1998)
Procyanidins extracted from pine bark protect a-tocopherol in ECV 304 endothelial cells challenged by activated RAW 264.7 macrophages: role of nitric oxide peroxynitrite.
FEBS letters, 431:315-318.

Wang, S., Tan, D. , Zhao, Y., Gao, G., Gao, X. and Hu, L. (1999)
The effect of Pycnogenol® on the microcirculation, platelet function and ischemic myocardium in patients with coronary artery diseases.
European Bulletin of Drug Research. 7 (2): 19-25.

Watson, R. (1999)
Reduction of cardiovascular disease risk factors by French Maritime Pine Bark Extract.
Cardiovascular Reviews and Reports XX (VI): 326-329.

Wei, Z H., Peng Q.L. and Lau B.H.S. (1997)
Pycnogenol® enhances endothelial cell antioxidant defences.
Redox Report, 3 (4): 219-224.

Yang TCT, Kaul, N. Devaraj. S. and Jialal, I.
The Effect of Pycnogenol®
Supplementation on Oxidative Stress.
FASEB J. **15(5)**: Part 2 A992 (Mar 8 2001)

106

SUGGESTED READINGS

Packer, L., Rimbach, G. and Virgili, F. (1999)
Antioxidant activity and biologic properties of a procyanidin-rich extract from the pine (Pinus maritima) bark, Pycnogenol.
Review Article In Free Radical Biology and Medicine, 27(5/6): 704-724.

Rohdewald, P. (1998)
Pycnogenol®.
In "Flavonoids in Health and Disease", ed. Catherine A. Rice-Evans and Lester Packer, *Marcel Dekker Inc. NY, 1998, Chapter 17, pages 405-419.*

Lynn, J.L.(1999)
Attention deficit Disorder, pages 1-31.
Pub.Impact communications, Inc. Green Bay, WI, USA.

Website http://www.pycnogenol.com

INDEX

A

ACE. See angiotension converting enzyme.
acute myocardial (heart) infarction. *See* heart
ADD, 81
ADHD, 81, 82, 85
adrenaline, 38, 39
aging, 10, 21, 22, 26, 59, 63, 73, 88
Aging, 59
Allergies, 78
Alzheimer's disease, 17, 18, 21, 26, 62
angina. *See* heart
angiotensin I converting enzyme, 36, 43, 44
apoptosis, 51
arteries, 10, 33, 34, 36, 37, 39, 42, 43, 46, 77
arthritis, 26, 49, 55, 56, 59
aspirin, 6, 8, 41
atherosclerosis. *See* heart
Atherosclerosis. *See* heart
Athletic Performance, 59
Attention deficit disorder, 81
Attention Deficit Hyperactivity Disorder, 81

B

bioflavonoids, 1, 2, 3, 4, 7, 9, 11, 14, 15, 24, 31, 52, 65
Blazso, 36, 37, 56, 67
blood cells, 10, 35, 36, 37, 46, 54, 66, 68
blood clots, 39, 47
blood platelets, 19, 36, 37, 38, 39, 40, 41, 44, 93, 95
blood pressure, 12, 34, 36, 38, 41, 42, 44, 45, 46, 59, 83
blood vessel, 35, 37, 38, 46
blood vessels, 4, 10, 11, 14, 33, 36, 38, 39, 40, 41, 42, 44, 47, 65, 66, 67
bruises, 65

C

CAM. *See* cellular adhesion molecules
cancer, 5, 22, 26, 49, 50, 51, 52, 53, 54, 59, 71, 78, 95
capillaries, 10, 11, 14, 48, 56, 65, 66, 67, 87
carcinogens, 50, 51, 52, 53

cataract, 26, 55, 71, 73
catechin, 2, 7, 23, 73
cellular adhesion molecules, 46, 97
chloasma. *See* melasma
cholesterol, 33, 34, 35, 36, 42
circulation, 5, 10, 33, 46, 47, 65, 68, 76, 84
collagen, 10, 11, 14, 37, 47, 87, 88
coronary thrombosis. *See* heart
cosmetic, 61, 87

D

Degenerative Diseases, 49
deoxyribonucleic acid. *See* DNA
diabetes, 38, 46, 49, 55, 72
DNA, 25, 50, 52, 53, 60, 95

E

Economy-Class Syndrome, 65, 68
edema, 56, 65, 66, 67
elastin, 10, 11, 47, 87
embolism, 38, 69
endometriosis, 76
endurance, 63
epicatechin, 2, 7, 23

exercise, 46, 63
eye, 26, 71, 72, 73

F

Fertility, 75
Fitzpatrick, 36, 39, 42, 44
French maritime pine tree, 4, 7

G

Gabor, 17, 45, 66, 67, 90
Gulati, 65, 76

H

HDL, 34
heart, 8, 10, 11, 17, 22, 26, 27, 33, 34, 36, 37, 38, 39, 41, 42, 43, 44, 46, 47, 48, 55, 69, 78, 97
Horphag Research, 15, 19, 93
hyperactivity, 81
hyperpigmentation, 90
hypertension. *See* blood pressure

I

immune system, 10, 12, 17, 18, 49, 50, 51, 52, 53, 54, 97
immunity, 53, 54
infarct.. *See* heart
infertility, 75, 76
inflammation, 36, 46, 55, 56, 78, 89, 90
inflammatory, 3, 5, 17, 18, 27, 46, 56, 57, 90

L

Lau, 18, 46, 53, 56, 63
LDL, 26, 34, 35, 37, 46
lifespan, 59, 61, 62
lupus, 26

M

Melasma, 90
memory, 18, 43, 63, 84
menses. *See* menstrual
menstrual, 5, 18, 75, 76

N

neuropathy, 55
NF-kB, 53
nitric oxide, 27, 36, 39, 40, 41, 42, 43, 44, 47, 48, 76, 77, 84, 97
Nuclear Factor-kappa B. *See* NF-kB

O

oligomeric procyanidins, 7, 29
oncogene, 50

P

Packer, 17, 27, 28, 42, 54, 56, 62, 90
Parkinson's disease, 21, 26
patent, 11, 16, 19, 93
petechiae, 66
Pinus maritima, 1, 7
Pinus pinaster, 1, 7
platelet. *See* blood platelet
platelet aggregation, 26, 33, 39, 40, 48
PMS, 75
proanthocyanidins, 4
procyanidins, 1, 2, 4, 5, 6, 7, 9, 15, 23, 24, 29
psoriasis, 26, 90

R

retinopathy, 18, 26, 55, 71, 72, 93
Rohdewald, 15, 17, 19, 39, 40, 41, 45, 89, 95

S

safety, 17, 95
scurvy, 2, 9, 11, 13, 14, 15, 87

112

Sexual Function, 75
skin, 8, 10, 11, 14, 17,
    26, 47, 61, 66, 67, 87,
    88, 89, 90
Skincare, 87
smoking, 11, 36, 38, 39
sperm, 26, 75
stress, 6, 10, 11, 36, 38,
    39, 60, 62, 93
stroke, 10, 12, 26, 38,
    39, 47, 69
Sunburn, 89
Systemic Lupus
    Erythematoses. *See*
    lupus
Szent-Gyorgyi, 3, 11,
    17, 66, 90

T

thrombus, 38, 47
trademark, 4, 19, 93
Trevithick, 73

V

varicose veins, 65, 67
Vasoconstriction, 34
vein, 10, 68
Venous, 65
vitamin C, 2, 3, 11, 14,
    15, 24, 27, 28, 30, 35,
    37, 52, 66, 72, 73, 75,
    94
vitamin E, 24, 27, 28, 29,
    30, 31, 35, 36, 37, 73,
    75

W

Wang, 48
Watson, 17, 39, 41, 45,
    47, 53, 54
Wei, 23, 42
Weight Control, 59
wrinkles, 61, 87

About the Author

Richard A. Passwater, Ph.D has published over 40 books and over 400 articles on nutrition, having been a research biochemist since 1959. His laboratory research led to his discovery of biological antioxidant synergism in 1962 which has been the focus of his research and patents ever since.

Dr. Passwater has been the Director of the Solgar Nutritional Research Center since 1979. Dr. Passwater is an independent researcher and author and does not consult for, nor is he in any way affiliated with, Horphag Research, the producer of the subject material, Pycnogenol®.

Dr. Passwater was the first to show that practical combinations of antioxidant nutrients increase the lifespan of laboratory animals (Chemical & Engineering News 1970).

Dr. Passwater was also the first to publish that a synergistic combination of antioxidant nutrients significantly reduce cancer incidence (Cancer: New Directions. American Laboratory 1973). Dr. Passwater was the first to publish an epidemiological study showing that vitamin E reduces heart disease risk (Prevention 1976).